ATHEROMA

Atherosclerosis in Ischaemic Heart Disease: Myocardial Consequences

Volume 2

P A Poole-Wilson MD FRCP
Professor of Cardiology
National Heart and Lung Insititute, London

D J Sheridan MD PhD FRCP
Professor of Cardiology
St Mary's Hospital, London

Presented as a service to cardiology
by Bayer UK Limited

Bayer C·A·R·E

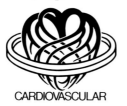

CARDIOVASCULAR

This book is Volume 2 of a two-volume series entitled *Atheroma*

Any product mentioned in this book should be used in accordance with the prescribing information prepared by the manufacturers. No claim or endorsement is made for any drug or compound presently under clinical investigation.

This book represents the findings of its authors and its contents do not necessarily reflect the opinion of Bayer UK Limited.

British Library Cataloguing in Publication Data
Atheroma
Vol 2
1. Man. Cardiovascular system. Diseases
I. Poole-Wilson P.A. (Philip Alexander) II. Sheridan D.J.
(Desmond John)
616.1

ISBN 1-870026-31-4
ISBN 1-870026-41-1 set
ISBN 1-870026-36-5 V.1

Edited by Sharyn Wong
Designed by Robin Dodd FCSD
Printed in Spain by Imago Publishing Limited

CONTENTS

3
The Myocardium in Ischaemic Heart Disease

The last twenty years have witnessed spectacular advances in the understanding and treatment of heart disease due to atheroma in the coronary arteries. Large population studies have provided key information on the epidemiology of coronary artery disease, leading to the identification of some of the factors associated with the development of atheroma. These risk factors have been used to detect, within a given population, those who are most likely to have a coronary event. The detection of early coronary disease, although still less than satisfactory, has been greatly aided by developments in exercise-testing, 24-hour monitoring of the electrocardiogram (ECG), echocardiography, Doppler flow measurements, magnetic resonance and radionuclide imaging. New treatments include advice on lifestyle, drugs to counter lipid abnormalities, thrombolytic and platelet drugs in acute myocardial infarction, drugs to delay the progression of myocardial dysfunction in heart failure, and the use of numerous drugs for the treatment of angina pectoris. Invasive treatments have also been expanded. Coronary artery bypass surgery is a successful operation for the treatment of angina pectoris and is now less dangerous through the use of cardioplegia. Percutaneous angioplasty (PTCA) has become a commonplace procedure.

Some ideas have proved to be erroneous while others have not fulfilled expectation. The benefit from preventive measures for myocardial infarction has been less than anticipated. Clinical trials have shown that some interventions, notably the administration of beta-blockers *(1-6)* or thrombolytic agents *(7-12)*, can reduce mortality after myocardial infarction, but the concept of altering 'infarct size' by preservation of the 'border zone' has been shown to be wrong *(13,14)*.

The advent of angioplasty *(15)* and thrombolytic therapy *(16-18)* for the treatment of events associated with atheromatous lesions in coronary arteries has reawakened interest in the causation of myocardial infarction and the early metabolic events following its onset. Several approaches to the early detection and treatment of coronary artery disease, such as public education, prevention clinics, cardiac resuscitation, coronary ambulances, coronary care units and thrombolysis, have contributed to a fall in mortality from coronary artery disease. This effect on acute mortality and, more importantly, on long-term mortality, would be greater if it were possible to delay the onset of tissue necrosis to allow more time for treatment to reduce the amount of necrosed myocardial muscle. Interventions may be developed to modify favourably the repair process and prevent infarct expansion (19).

Understanding the metabolic changes in early ischaemia is also relevant to the genesis of arrhythmias and sudden death, which accounts for a large proportion of deaths due to coronary artery disease before reaching hospital and in the absence of medical expertise (20).

Epidemiology and the clinical problem

Coronary artery disease is manifest in man as angina pectoris, myocardial infarction, sudden death or heart failure. It is the most common cause of death in men aged 45 to 65 years in Western countries and accounts for almost 50% of deaths. Death from myocardial infarction often occurs (50% of cases) within six hours after the onset of chest pain (20). Thus, as the opportunity to reduce mortality by acute interventions is always limited, prevention is an important approach.

The incidence of death due to coronary artery disease varies between countries (21,22) (Figures 3.1 and 3.2) and between genders. There is a much greater variation in men than in

Figure 3.1 Coronary heart disease mortality in 1985 for men and women aged between 40 and 60 years (age standardized). Note that the mortality for women is very much lower than that for men. For men, there is a wide variation between countries. From Tunstall-Pedoe, *Br Med J* 1989; **298**: 751.

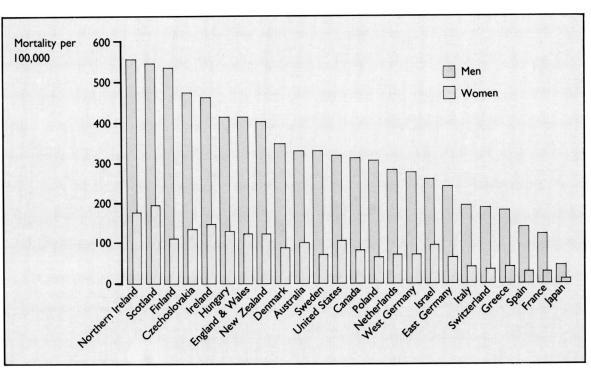

women and, in women, it occurs at a later age, after the menopause. Many of these differences between countries are real, but a substantial proportion may represent differences in the diagnosis of and social attitudes towards ischaemic heart disease in these countries *(23)*. In the UK, for example, sudden death in an elderly person is often officially attributed to ischaemic heart disease, although such a diagnosis may be difficult to demonstrate at post mortem even if such a procedure is undertaken. As many as 40% of sudden deaths are not attributable to coronary heart disease *(24)*. Ischaemic heart disease is often the destitute, but socially acceptable, diagnosis of the physician. Likewise, the difference between death due to heart failure and death due to coronary artery disease can be confusing. With increasing interest in heart failure, some deaths which would previously have been attributed to coronary artery disease may now be considered cardiac failure.

Numerous studies have shown that certain so-called 'risk factors' are linked to an increased probability of death from coronary artery disease *(25-27)*. Many of these risk factors are more correctly considered 'associations' as they are either unalterable or, when changed, have not been shown to reduce the incidence of coronary events (as required by use of the word 'risk'). A risk can be avoided, but an association cannot.

Figure 3.2 Coronary artery disease (CAD) mortality (in 1980) in different countries related to serum cholesterol. Although there is a relationship, there is considerable variation. Note the differences between the United States, England & Wales and France despite similar cultural habits. Adapted from Simons, *Am J Cardiol* 1986; **57**: 5-10G.

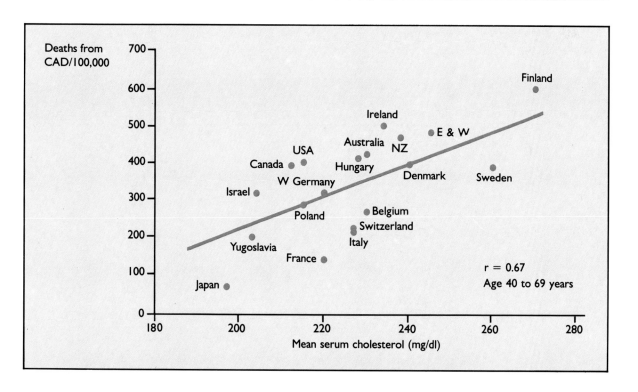

Often, the risk factor may be a marker of the disease rather than a causal agent. There is also the possibility of mistaking a correlation of two variables as proof of a causal relationship; for example, the increased incidence of coronary artery disease in this century correlates with the introduction of central heating and the alteration of many social habits. A tantalizing correlation recently described *(28)* is that between mortality from ischaemic heart disease and geographical latitude (Figure 3.3).

The most significant risk factors are male gender, age and a family history. These are unalterable, as may be others such as personality and some forms of behaviour. Those risk factors which can be manipulated and most closely predict coronary artery disease are hypertension, lipid abnormalities, carbohydrate abnormalities (diabetes) and cigarette-smoking. Obesity and a sedentary lifestyle are of less significance.

> Over 50% of coronary events can be predicted from a simple assessment of risk factors in individuals from the general population *(29)*. Put another way, as many as 46% of patients have coronary heart disease which cannot be explained by current risk factors. This is particularly true for women in whom there is an increase in the importance of coronary artery disease after the menopause.

Even if the assessment of risk on the basis of risk factors indicates a high relative risk, the absolute risk for those in the worst categories is modest. The Pooling Project *(26)* indicated that men aged 45 to 49 at entry and in the top 20% for risk had an 8% chance of a coronary event in 8.6 years. They estimated that two-thirds of men aged 40 to 55 years in the worst 20%

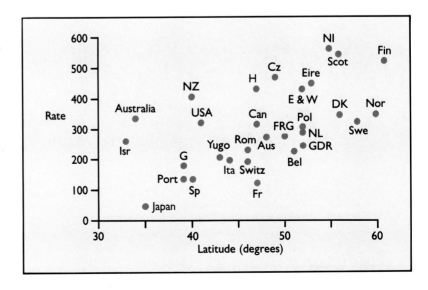

Figure 3.3 Ischaemic heart disease mortality ratio in different countries plotted against latitude. There appears to be a relationship. The reason is contentious. *From reference 28*

for risk factors were likely to be fit 25 years later. An analysis from a different group of workers *(30)*, using a model incorporating multiple risk factors, calculated that for persons at high risk, the gain in life expectancy from a dietary programme was between 18 days and one year. Furthermore, it is not proven that all of these risk factors are reversible causes of coronary artery disease *(31)* (Table 3.1). Most notably, the treatment of hypertension has not been shown to lead to a reduction in the incidence of coronary events (Tables 3.2 and 3.3) *(32-42)*.

The role of lipid abnormalities in the causation of heart disease and the benefits of treatment are still subjects of controversy *(43-46)*. For over a decade, the topic has been forcefully discussed *(31,47-51)* and strong views expressed; little has changed *(44,46)*.

The nature of the controversy is often misunderstood.

Most physicians would agree that advice and attention to cigarette-smoking, obesity, diet, hypertension and exercise is appropriate for those with coronary artery disease *(52)*. Indeed, such a multifactorial approach to the prevention of disease is appropriate for almost the entire population.

Table 3.1   Interventional trials in coronary heart disease..

			CHD deaths		Total deaths		% Reduction		
Trial	Size	Years	Int	Plac	Int	Plac	CHD	Total	Lives Saved/ 1000 treated
Multiple interventions									
WHO	60 881	6	428	450	1 325	1 341	5	1	0.5
Göteborg	30 000	12	462	461	1 293	1 318	0	1.9	1.7
MRFIT	12 866	7	115	124	265	260	7	+2	−0.8
Helsinki	1 222	5	4	4	10	5	0	+50	−8
Oslo	1 232	5	6	13	16	23	54	30	11
Cholesterol									
WHO (clof)	15 745	5	54	48	162	127	+13	+28	−4
LRC-CPPT	3 806	7	32	44	68	71	27	4	1.6
Gemfibrozil	4 081	5	6	8	45	42	25	+7	−1.5
Smoking									
Whitehall	1 445	10	49	62	123	128	21	4	7
Hypertension									
8 trials	17 314	−	−	−	784	887	−	12	12
MRC	17 354	5	106	97	248	253	+9	2	0.6

From McCormick and Skrabanek, *Lancet* 1988; ii: 839 Int = Intervention Plac = Placebo

Table 3.2   Trials of treatment in mild hypertension

	Total mortality	Stroke mortality	n	CHD mortality Control	CHD mortality Treated
VA	?↓	?↓	380	12	6
Göteborg	?↓		635	6	
HDFP	?↓	?↓	10940	69 (148)	51 (131)
Oslo		↓	785	2	6
Australian	?↓	↓	3427	11	5
MRFIT			8011	79	80
European			840	47	29
IPPPSH			6357	46	40
MRC		↓	17354	97	106
HEP		↓	884	25	28
HAPPHY			6567	50	54

Such simple advice is not recognized sufficiently by the public because of debate and argument over the role of lipids and, in particular, cholesterol *(43-51)*. The evangelists may have done harm by delaying the introduction of changes in lifestyle in the general population through encouraging the perception that the medical profession is in disarray.

> The debate over the interpretation of data and the most appropriate way to implement change cannot be decided or decreed by consensus conferences or committees. These merely influence thinking and any indication of bias by such groups may result in a loss of credibility. Many physicians are arguing that the results of recent trials have been promulgated in an overly optimistic or even misleading manner *(43,45)*.

Table 3.3   Trials of treatment in mild hypertension

Trial	Year	Sex	Age	Blood pressure	n	Type
VA	1970	M	51	90–114	380	R,D
Göteborg	1978	M	47–54	175/115	635	–
HDFP	1979	M,F	30–69	>90	10940	R
Oslo	1980	M	40–49	150–179/>10	785	R
Australian	1980	M,F	30–69	95–109	3427	R,S
MRFIT	1982	M	35–59	90–115	12866	R
European	1985	M,F	over 60	90–119	840	R,D
IPPPSH	1985	M,F	40–69	100–125	6357	R,D
MRC	1985	M,F	35–60	90–109	17354	R,S
HEP	1986	M,F	60–79	170/105	884	R
HAPPHY	1987	M	40–64	100–130	6569	R

R = Randomized; D = Double-blind; S = Single-blind

Figure 3.4 Age-adjusted mortality over six years per 10,000 men aged 35 to 57 years shows that the total number of deaths in CAD increases with the serum cholesterol levels, and is also higher for the lower levels of cholesterol. Over the middle range of serum cholesterol, the change in total deaths is small. From MRFIT, *N Engl J Med* 1989; **320**: 904.

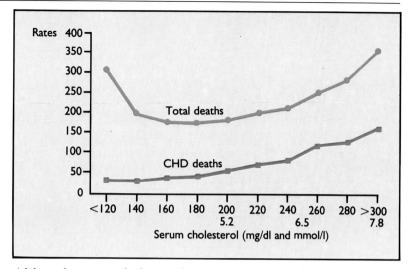

Although serum cholesterol concentration is related to the occurrence of death from coronary artery disease (Figure 3.4), it is not well related to death from all causes *(53)*. Indeed, there is a suspicion that a low plasma cholesterol is associated with an increased mortality (54). This has been attributed to the presence of undiagnosed illness, such as cancer. The low cholesterol, it is suggested, is a marker of disease and thus associated with an increased mortality. This explanation cannot account for the fact that the relationship is still present if all deaths in the early years after the measurement of cholesterol concentration are ignored. A further point to note is that the relationship between coronary deaths and cholesterol is not linear (Figure 3.4). Therefore, if alteration of the cholesterol in a group of patients moved that population along the curve shown in Figure 3.4 (an assumption which is probably correct), the higher the initial cholesterol concentration, the greater the number of persons benefiting. For those with a cholesterol concentration below 6 mmol/l, the number of deaths prevented is small.

Evidence from several sources has shown that coronary events may be prevented by lowering the plasma cholesterol, thus supporting the lipid hypothesis of atheroma. Three drug trials *(55-57)* (Table 3.4) have shown a reduction in coronary events, but not in total deaths. The most persuasive evidence is the relationship between the reduction of cholesterol achieved in trials and the reduction of coronary events (Figure 3.5). In one trial *(58)* in patients following coronary artery bypass surgery, the progression of lesions in native vessels was reduced, new atheroma was less, and new or adverse changes in grafts were reduced. A more recent study *(59)* indicates that a calcium antagonist, nifedipine, may reduce the development of new atherosclerotic lesions in patients who already have atheroma of the coronary arteries.

Several large trials have not provided the anticipated evidence of benefit from manipulation of risk factors *(25,26,60)*.

Table 3.4   Lipid intervention trials

	Cholesterol reduction (%)	n		Cardiac events		Cardiac deaths		Total deaths	
		Plac	Rx	Plac	Rx	Plac	Rx	Plac	Rx
WHO Clofibrate	8	5296	5331	208	167	34	36	59	54
LRC Cholestyramine	9	1900	1906	187	155 (p<0.05)	38	30	71	68
Helsinki Gemfibrozil	9	2030	2051	72	46 (p<0.02)	19	14	42	45
Total		9226	9228	467 (−21%)	368	91 (−12%)	80	172 (−3%)	167

Plac = Placebo; Rx = Active treatment.

This may be because the subjects were middle-aged men, the duration was too short (five years), patients in the control group also altered their lifestyles, or the original hypothesis was wrong. The Framingham study reported a 30-year follow-up *(27)*. Blood cholesterol concentrations were found to be related to total mortality in men under the age of 50 years at the start of the study. This is the first demonstration of a key part of the controversy, namely, whether total mortality is related to blood cholesterol concentrations, and contrasts with shorter studies (Tables 3.1 and 3.4). No relationship was observed in persons over 50 years of age at the beginning of the study. An unexplained finding was that those who had a fall in cholesterol concentrations in the first 14 years of the follow-up had an increased total mortality and death from coronary artery disease. Not all of the results are understood.

It may be that a major impact on the development of atheroma requires treatment to begin at a young age. Follow-up for more than five years is needed to demonstrate any effect. Furthermore, coronary events are probably related to other phenomena, such as platelet function, endothelial cell function and circulating clotting factors, which precipitate a coronary event when atheroma is present. In effect, a high serum cholesterol concentration may be a factor in determining the development of atheroma, but only as a substrate and not as a trigger for coronary events.

The major difficulties with the dietary approach to the treatment of coronary artery disease are public resistance to change of dietary habits, the expense, whether only advice is given

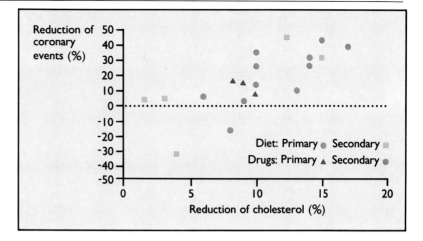

Figure 3.5 Twenty various trials plotted to show reduction of coronary events against reduction of cholesterol. The resulting picture provides some evidence of an association between serum cholesterol and death from CAD.

or drugs prescribed, and the large number of individuals who need to be advised in order to gain advantage for a few *(39,49-51)*. This approach to prevention is costly and inefficient. New methods for the early identification of coronary artery disease linked to advice for those at greatest risk may prove to be a more effective policy.

Experimental ischaemia

The normal heart

The limiting substrate for the heart is oxygen. The heart is dependent on a controlled and variable flow of blood in the coronary arteries to supply oxygen to the muscle. The normal human heart weighs approximately 300 g. Coronary blood flow at rest is 0.8 ml^{-1}.g^{-1}. Arterial blood contains 188 ml.l^{-1} of oxygen (arterial PO_2 = 100 mmHg and the blood is 98% saturated with oxygen). The oxygen content of blood in the coronary sinus is substantially lower than that of mixed venous blood (in the pulmonary artery), being 68 ml.l^{-1} (coronary venous PO_2 = 25 mmHg and the blood is 30% saturated with oxygen). Simple calculation shows that the resting oxygen consumption of the heart is 27 ml.min^{-1} or 0.09 ml.min^{-1}.g^{-1}. The resting cardiac output of the heart in an average person is 5 l.min^{-1}, which increases on exercise to 25 l.min^{-1} or more. This fivefold increase in cardiac output results from a threefold increase in heart rate and a lesser increase in stroke volume.

In contrast to other tissues and, in particular, skeletal muscle, the availability of oxygen in the heart can be increased to only a limited extent as a result of a widening of the arteriovenous difference (greater extraction). When heart rate increases in a normal heart, there is a transient fall in the oxygen content in the coronary sinus for approximately 15 seconds. During this time, the coronary resistance falls. Increased availability of oxygen to the heart is provided by an increased coronary blood flow, rather than increased extraction, which may increase by as much as four times. With increasing heart rate, the proportion of time that the heart is in systole (when little blood flows to the myocardium) increases. Thus, the true resistance to blood flow, the pressure-flow relationship in diastole, must be reduced proportionally more than the overall increase in blood flow. In the presence of a severe stenosis in the coronary arteries, coronary sinus oxygen falls and remains low – an indication of ischaemia *(61)*.

The major determinant of blood flow in the coronary arteries is myocardial oxygen consumption (metabolic regulation; Figure 3.6). Coronary blood flow is maintained almost as a constant over a wide range of diastolic blood pressure (autoregulation). Neural and hormonal mechanisms are secondary control mechanisms of coronary blood flow to the heart *(62,63)*.

Figure 3.6 Coronary flow plotted against coronary perfusion pressure. At normal or low workload levels, there is little variation over a considerable range of perfusion pressure (autoregulation). At a given coronary perfusion pressure, flow increases greatly with the workload (metabolic regulation).

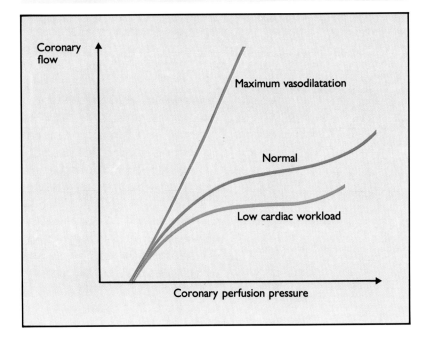

The mechanisms underlying metabolic control and autoregulation of the heart are poorly understood. Endothelium-derived relaxing factor (EDRF) may have an important role in pathological conditions *(64)* and, under normal conditions, may control and maintain an even distribution of blood flow through the multiple arteries supplying the myocardium. When the endothelium is damaged or absent, instead of vasodilatation of the coronary arteries due to the release of EDRF, many substances cause vasoconstriction by a direct effect on the smooth muscle.

Why the coronary sinus oxygen content is maintained at a constant over a wide range of oxygen consumption by the heart is not known. It may be that the oxygen partial pressure in the capillaries is optimal and provides a maximum flux of oxygen into the cells. Furthermore, it is not clear how the tight relationship between increased cardiac work, stimulation of metabolism and increased coronary blood flow is controlled. An elevated cytosolic calcium is one possible signal relating contraction to metabolism. Coronary blood flow is influenced by pH, K^+, adenosine and other factors which are metabolites likely to accumulate in ischaemia.

Definition of ischaemia

Ischaemia is often defined as a state in which an imbalance between oxygen supply and demand is present (Table 3.5). Although such a definition, when applied to the heart, has great conceptual appeal to the clinician, its practical value is minimal as it is difficult, if not impossible, to measure directly both these entities in intact man. Metabolic poisoning, in which there is a clear imbalance between so-called supply and demand, would be regarded as ischaemia. Furthermore, such a definition is an incorrect use of language. The heart does not demand oxygen, nor is the sole function of the coronary circulation to provide oxygen. The removal of metabolites, notably heat and acid in the form of carbon dioxide, is as important a function of myocardial blood flow as is the supply of substrate (glucose and fat) and oxygen.

Table 3.5 Definition of ischaemia
Traditional
Imbalance in the supply and demand of oxygen
Alternative
Non-steady state of high-energy phosphate turnover
Detect by:
Lactate production;
Acidosis;
Venous oxygen saturation

A more useful definition of ischaemia is that it is an imbalance between the rate of adenosine triphosphate (ATP) consumption and blood flow. Ischaemia arises either when ATP consumption increases above the rate of ATP production sustainable by a given blood flow, or when blood flow is so reduced that the existing rate of ATP consumption cannot be maintained.

In the first minute of ischaemia, flux through the glycolytic pathway is greatly stimulated (Pasteur effect), but is subsequently inhibited by the development of an acidosis and the accumulation of citrate, reduced nicotinamide-adenine dinucleotide (NADH) and lactate *(65-67)*. The available oxygen is insufficient to permit oxidative phosphorylation, and pyruvate (the end-product of the glycolytic chain), instead of passing into the Kreb's cycle, is converted to lactic acid.

Ischaemia can be defined more simply as a state characterized by the flow-related accumulation of lactic acid or hydrogen ions, or flow-related maximum extraction of oxygen from arterial blood.

A major advantage of such a definition is that methods are readily available for the detection of ischaemia. Lactate measurement in the coronary sinus particularly during atrial pacing has been used for many years. Alternatively, pH *(68)* can be measured in the coronary sinus using continuously recording electrodes. A fall of coronary sinus oxygen is another sensitive indicator of ischaemia. Coronary sinus oxygen falls immediately in spontaneous angina *(69)* or when angina is induced by atrial pacing *(61)*.

Modish terms in current use
There has, in the last few years, been a proliferation of new words and phrases applied to the ischaemic myocardium. Some have been coined to dramatize clinical syndromes associated with the ischaemic myocardium, some to characterize ideas relating to pathophysiology, and others to popularize concepts linked to certain experimental models and the consequences of reperfusion (see Box).

> New words and phrases applicable to ischaemic myocardium include: Reversible and irreversible damage; jeopardized myocardium; threatened myocardium; lethal ischaemia; border zone; salvaged myocardium; infarct size; area at risk.
>
> More recent examples (Table 3.6) are: Stunned myocardium *(70)*; stuttering ischaemia *(71)*; hibernating myocardium *(202)*; mummified myocardium *(72)*; ischaemic preconditioning; total ischaemic burden *(73)*.

Table 3.6 Fashionable terms for myocardial damage

Stunned myocardium

Hibernating myocardium

Mummified myocardium

Stuttering ischaemia

Preconditioning

Chronic ischaemia

Ischaemic cardiomyopathy

Some of these latter phrases are used in much the same sense as the earlier concept of 'chronic ischaemia' or the disputed phrase 'ischaemic cardiomyopathy'.

Such jargon is a useful 'shorthand' for the exchange of ideas between investigators and physicians and, thus, has become acceptable in the cardiological literature. Often the phrases give a spurious scientific credibility to ideas which are not always proven or supported by experimental evidence. Many are poorly defined, if at all. Stunned myocardium *(70)* exists when, after a short period of ischaemia, recovery of mechanical function is incomplete, but there is no cell necrosis. Such a definition is applicable to the dog, in which it is possible to perform detailed histological examination of the myocardium, but not in man, in whom it cannot be demonstrated whether the duration of ischaemia is so brief that necrosis has not occurred. Hibernating myocardium *(202)* is a state where, in the presence of coronary artery disease, myocardial function is reduced and can be improved by revascularization. Thus, it is almost akin to persistence of stunned myocardium. The use of phrases which attribute human or animal characteristics ('stunned', 'hibernating', 'alive' and 'dead') to pieces of muscle is not illuminating.

An important example of how confusion may be generated is the overuse of the distinction implied by the use of the phrases 'reversible' and 'irreversible' to describe damage during ischaemia.

Such a concept is almost wholly misleading. Whether the myocardium has been irreversibly damaged can only be established by reperfusion of the myocardium and later quantitation of the amount of necrotic tissue. Myocardium which is not reperfused dies; that is a truism. There is no means of characterizing myocytes as irreversibly damaged during ischaemia as key events may occur at the moment of reperfusion and an intervention may arise which can reduce the amount of subsequent necrotic tissue. It is not possible to distinguish reversible and irreversible damage before reperfusion if the sole criterion is the response to reperfusion. The only exception to this argument is total loss of cell organization or disruption of the sarcolemma during ischaemia, but the dispute is then trivial since, under such circumstances, all tissue is unquestionably irreversibly damaged. Such damage is a late event and a statement of the obvious is not useful to the experimentalist or clinician.

Models of ischaemia
The consequences of ischaemia or hypoxia have been studied in many experimental situations including sarcolemmal vesicles, single isolated cells, papillary muscles, Langendorff perfused hearts, working isolated hearts, intact conscious or unconscious dogs and, more recently, rabbits and rats. These models were selected to provide answers to questions which may advance understanding of the events during ischaemia. No model is ideal and all have important limitations.

Sudden occlusion of a coronary artery by external compression in a dog with an extensive collateral blood supply of congenital origin is not equivalent to the onset of myocardial infarction in man. Myocardial infarction is often due to thrombus formation preceded by repetitive episodes of transient ischaemia due to platelet aggregation on a vessel wall damaged by the recent disruption of an atheromatous plaque *(74,75)*. However, a collateral blood supply may have developed over many years in response to ischaemic episodes. The dog model has often been considered an appropriate substitute for man because of the presence of collaterals in contrast to other species, such as the rabbit, but collaterals of genetic origin may be different from collaterals which have developed in response to repeated episodes of ischaemia.

Species differences are common and may point to important factors determining infarct size; for example, dogs and rats have xanthine oxidase in their heart tissue whereas the rabbit has none and man little, making the activity of this enzyme (76) of little importance in the generation of radicals in the human myocardium.

Differences between models of myocardial ischaemia can be revealing. Recent reports, for example, suggest that, early in ischaemia, the myocardium becomes transiently alkalotic (77-79) and not acidotic (80,81). The alkalosis is the result of breakdown of creatine phosphate (CP). If this observation were applicable to man, then acidosis, which all workers agree develops later in ischaemia, cannot be contributory to the early decline of contractile function. Yet, in man, acidosis can be detected after only 15 seconds of ischaemia during coronary occlusion in patients undergoing angioplasty (68). This is the first moment that contractile abnormalities can be detected in man (82). The probable reason for these differences is that, in man *in vivo*, the oxygen consumption of the heart is so much greater that acidosis from the breakdown of ATP counterbalances the consumption of hydrogen ions due to the metabolism of CP. Reduction in temperature, heart rate and oxygen consumption in experimental models has demonstrated the presence of an important phenomenon, namely, alkalosis, which does not occur in intact man.

Cytosolic ionic concentrations have been measured during ischaemia and hypoxia under conditions where resting tension in the myocardium increases only marginally, or increases but can be rapidly and easily reversed in contrast to similar mechanical changes in intact models. The reported changes in cytosolic ion concentrations may have little relevance to those changes which occur at the moment of reperfusion which result in cell damage. In the absence of a rise in resting tension, reperfusion almost always results in full recovery of contractile function and no net gain of calcium (83).

> The limitations of experimental models must be appreciated, and invidious comparison between models is a destructive debate.

Biochemistry of myocardial ischaemia

Early changes. After total occlusion of a coronary artery, there is sufficient oxygen in the myocardium to supply energy for two to three heart beats (84). High-energy phosphates (ATP and CP) within the myocardium may provide energy for a further six to 10 beats. The total tissue ATP level does not fall for several minutes whereas the tissue content of CP falls so rapidly that, by the end of two to three minutes, it has been reduced by almost 80% *(85-87)*. Creatine phosphate is believed to be, in part, an energy reserve system within the heart muscle, providing immediate energy for contraction by donating its high-energy phosphate group to adenosine diphosphate (ADP) to produce ATP and creatine.

Myocardial contractility declines rapidly and almost ceases within 90 seconds *(88,89)*. In patients, changes in the surface ECG are detectable after approximately 30 seconds, and chest pain is experienced after 60 seconds. More recent studies have shown that the monophasic action potential is altered after approximately 16 heart beats *(90)*, when both contraction and relaxation of heart muscle are also modified *(82)*. It is difficult to evaluate the function of the whole heart as that is determined by the sum of regional abnormalities of contraction. During systole, ischaemic muscle develops a reduced tension and becomes stretched by the interventricular pressure generated by normal myocardial tissue. In addition, contraction of ischaemic muscle may be more prolonged than normal muscle, leading to incoordinated contraction and relaxation.

The mechanisms of many of these events have been established, although there is still some controversy. Several causes have been put forward for the early failure of myocardial contraction.

An immediate consequence of coronary artery occlusion is a loss of turgor in the artery. Pressure in the arteries of the heart splints and distends myocardial tissue, and removal of this effect leads to a reduction in sarcomere length and a fall in contractility.

This effect is known as the 'erectile' or 'garden-hose' effect *(92,93)*, and is accentuated in isolated muscle preparations perfused at high flow rates with physiological fluids. However, it appears to be a less important mechanism in man. The consequences of this phenomenon are evident within two to three heart beats.

The decline in the development of systolic tension beginning at around the sixteenth beat has other causes. It has variously been ascribed to intracellular acidosis, an accumulation of phosphate, accumulation of magnesium and a lack of energy for contraction *(91)*. For an explanation to be tenable, the putative factor must change sufficiently early and be of sufficient magnitude. Although, under some experimental conditions, the contractile tension can be shown to fall in the absence of an acidosis during ischaemia *(78)*, the fall of developed tension is usually accompanied by a drop in pH *(80,81)*.

In intact dogs, the acidosis is evident within fewer than 20 seconds *(94)* and more recent observations *(68)* show this to be true in man.

Several hypotheses have been proposed to account for the acidosis. During early ischaemia, oxygen in the tissue is converted to carbon dioxide, the glycolytic pathway is stimulated and lactate is generated from the small amount of glucose within the tissue and from tissue stores of glycogen. Because of the lack of oxygen, oxidative phosphorylation cannot proceed and citrate increases in the tissue. The increase of citrate and fall in ATP levels stimulate the enzyme phosphofructokinase in the glycolytic pathway to increase the glycolytic flux (the Pasteur effect). After approximately 30 seconds of ischaemia, glycolysis is reduced because acidosis inhibits the activity of phosphofructokinase and because acidosis, lactate and the accumulation of NADH inhibit the activity of glyceraldehyde-3-phosphate dehydrogenase, a more distal enzyme in the pathway.

> The generation of lactic acid and conversion of oxygen to carbon dioxide are probably the major causes for the early development of acidosis.

Early in ischaemia, the tissue content of ATP does not fall *(85-87)* and this cannot be a source of protons. The conversion of CP to creatine absorbs a proton and, under some circumstances, a transient alkalosis has been reported which, however, does not appear during ischaemia in the intact animal *(94)* or man *(68)*. Thus, acidosis occurs sufficiently early to explain some of the early reduction in developed tension.

The mechanisms by which acidosis reduces contraction is less certain. Acidosis is known to effect the transport of calcium across the sarcolemma, alter the slow calcium current, effect the uptake of calcium by the sarcoplasmic reticulum and alter the interaction of calcium with the contractile proteins. Recent work has shown that, during an imposed acidosis, the cytosolic calcium level increases *(95)*, suggesting that the major reason for the negative inotropic effect of an acidosis in the heart is a direct effect on the contractile proteins.

Another cause of early contractile failure is the accumulation of tissue phosphate *(96)* and possibly magnesium *(97)*. The breakdown of CP early in ischaemia leads to the accumulation of phosphate within the tissue *(96)*. Experiments on isolated muscle show that a raised cytosolic phosphate level reduces the contractile function of isolated myocardial fibres *(98)*.

The substance directly providing energy for contraction of the myocardium is ATP. The tissue content of ATP does not fall early during ischaemia *(85-87)* although, as CP levels do fall, it has been argued that ATP in the tissue is compartmentalized and that the ATP providing energy for contraction is diminished *(86)*. This hypothesis remains contentious and unproven *(99,100)*. The energy for contraction does not depend solely on the amount of ATP in the tissue, but also on the concentration of the end-products of the reaction. It is the free energy of the reaction that is critical to muscle function *(101,102)*. The increase in phosphate and ADP in the ischaemic tissue reduces the free energy available for contraction. Free energy is decreased early in ischaemia at the same time as contraction is reduced; the two have been related, although the causal link is in dispute *(101,102)*.

> The second major consequence of acute myocardial ischaemia is an alteration in the configuration of the action potential and the development of arrhythmias leading to clinical sudden death.

Changes in the conduction velocity, rate of depolarization, resting membrane potential and action-potential duration can be accounted for by known changes in pH and extracellular potassium *(103)*. Using potassium-sensitive electrodes, several groups *(103-108)* have recently shown that, soon after the onset of ischaemia, there is an accumulation of potassium in the extracellular space. The loss of potassium is rapid, occurring almost instantaneously in isolated tissues. In man, potassium loss is evident after around the sixteenth heart beat *(109)*. The extracellular potassium reaches a concentration of approximately 9 mmol.l^{-1} after three minutes and, after 15 minutes, reaches a concentration of 16 mmol.l^{-1}, which is retained for up to 25 minutes.

Subsequently, there is a further rise in the extracellular potassium concentration which may reach 40 mmol.l^{-1}. This secondary rise is thought to be due to destruction of myocardial cells and efflux of intracellular potassium. The early rise of potassium must have a different explanation because, if the tissue is reperfused, tissue function returns to normal and the myocardium takes up potassium, thus restoring the loss during the period of ischaemia. The timing and magnitude of the change in extracellular potassium is sufficient to account for alterations in the configuration of the action potential and other electrophysiological effects, particularly if the change in pH is taken into account *(103)*.

Several mechanisms have been put forward to account for the early loss of potassium. The loss is not due to a reduced influx of potassium, but to an increased efflux *(107,110)*. The sodium pump has been shown to be functional, if inhibited *(107,111)*, and the intracellular sodium activity of the myocardium is not changed for at least the initial 15 minutes of ischaemia *(112)*. The loss of potassium may be accounted for in part by the outward movement of permeant anions, such as lactate and phosphate *(110)*, which accumulate rapidly in the ischaemic myocardium, and in part due to alterations in membrane permeability to potassium, particularly during the action potential.

A potassium channel has been described which is sensitive to ATP and opens when ATP is reduced (113). Whether such a channel is associated with the loss of potassium is not yet known because of difficulties in establishing the concentrations of ATP in proximity to the cell membrane.

Late changes. Many biochemical changes take place in the myocardial cell during prolonged ischaemia. In the dog subjected to total ischaemia, little recovery of myocardial function occurs if the tissue is reperfused after 40 minutes *(114)*, a state which has been described as 'irreversibly' damaged *(115)*. In general, it is not possible to determine whether damage is irreversible except by reperfusion of the myocardium. However, many events occur at the time of reperfusion (see Box) and it is probable *(71)* that the degree of recovery may be altered by manipulation of conditions at the time of reperfusion. There is at present no method of ascertaining whether muscle is irreversibly damaged during a period of ischaemia except when gross disruption of the cell membrane is present.

Study of the cell function during ischaemia has shown that, by approximately 30 minutes of total global ischaemia, ATP concentration in the cell has fallen substantially *(114)*. Abnormalities can be demonstrated, under the electron microscope, in the function of the sarcoplasmic reticulum, mitochondria and cell membrane; lipids accumulate within the myocardial cell; mitochondrial swelling and aggregation of nuclear chromatin are early changes.

At about 30 minutes, the myofibrils shorten ('contracture' or 'rigor'), probably due to low ATP concentrations rather than an increased cytosolic calcium concentration. Myofibril shortening is a feature of total global myocardial ischaemia. In regional low-flow myocardial ischaemia, the myofibrils tend to be pulled apart by the contraction of adjacent normal muscle. Eventually, blebs form in the cell membrane *(117,118)*, discontinuities develop and gross disruption follows.

Changes in ion concentration within the myocardial cell during prolonged ischaemia are not well described. There is an early loss of potassium which later increases when cells are disrupted. Intracellular sodium does not accumulate for at least 15 minutes *(112)* and, although the sodium pump may be inhibited, it has been demonstrated to be functional *(107,111,112)*. Cytosolic calcium concentration appears to rise early (see Table 3.11) *(119,123)*.

Phospholipases are activated in the cell membrane, but gross changes in the lipids of the cell membrane appear to be a feature of late ischaemia *(124)*.

During total and global ischaemia, it is self-evident that there can be no change in the total tissue content of ions or of any other non-metabolizable substance. Such a situation rarely arises in man and is almost unknown in dogs. Collateral flow results in residual flow even at the centre of the infarcted muscle *(125,126)* and, in the presence of a continuing low flow, ion exchange can occur and there is a loss of enzymes. These enzymes are used as a marker of myocardial infarction by the clinician.

Reperfusion, recanalization and reflow

Table 3.7 Myocardial ischaemia: 'Reperfusion damage'

Transient increase of resting tension

Release of intracellular enzymes

Cell-swelling

Cell morphological/mitochondrial damage

Calcium accumulation

Transient loss of ion homeostasis

Recovery of energy production

Reperfusion is always beneficial

Reperfusion of heart muscle after more than 20 minutes of ischaemia is associated with the release of intracellular enzymes, a transient rise of resting tension, persisting functional abnormalities, influx of calcium, disruption of cell membranes and eventual necrosis of at least a proportion of the tissue.

This entity has been called reperfusion damage (Table 3.7) as much of the damage is believed to be the consequence of events occurring at the moment of reperfusion rather than a result of biochemical changes during the period of ischaemia. The early literature has been reviewed *(127)*.

Reperfusion of coronary arteries is usually achieved experimentally by release of some form of constrictor. Such rapid reperfusion is more harmful to the myocardium than slow restoration of flow *(128)*. In man in the context of myocardial infarction, the process is more complex and can be intermittent *(129,130)* – stuttering ischaemia. Ischaemia may be terminated either by natural thrombolysis or thrombolytic therapy.

The presence of coronary artery patency should not be confused with reperfusion.

Following a short period of ischaemia, flow is increased (the hyperaemic response). After more prolonged ischaemia, flow on release of the occlusion is greatly reduced, the so-called no-reflow phenomenon (131-135). If the myocardium is maximally vasodilated before ischaemia, then both ischaemia and hypoxia increase coronary resistance progressively (132). The increase of flow after short periods of ischaemia only arises because of initial tone in the coronary arteries. Many mechanisms contribute to the increase in resistance. Initially, the effect can be inhibited by calcium antagonists, suggesting that smooth muscle contraction is a factor (136). Later, resistance may be increased due to extravascular forces, such as myocardial oedema (137) and contracture of myocytes (138), plugging of arterioles (139), oedema of endothelial cells and endothelial damage. Haemorrhage may occur in dogs following sudden restoration of flow, but appears to be a rare event in man.

Existence of reperfusion damage
The existence of reperfusion damage has been challenged. Three arguments have been put forward. The first argument suggests that the markers of damage may merely be the 'washout' of metabolites and enzymes which accumulated during ischaemia and could only be detected when flow was restored. This argument is not strong as a similar phenomenon is observed on reoxygenation after low-flow ischaemia or a period of hypoxia (140) during which coronary flow is maintained constant. This is not to deny that such a washout of both potassium (109) and hydrogen ions (68) can be demonstrated in man on coronary artery occlusion during angioplasty.

The second argument is that the phenomenon is merely the evidence of necrosis of cells already completely destroyed during the period of ischaemia, and third, it has been suggested that the events on reperfusion are the abrupt expression of events which would inevitably become manifest over time. Changes in the cell during ischaemia inevitably lead to necrosis and abrupt reperfusion compresses that process into a short time span. According to this argument, alteration of events at the moment of reperfusion merely *delay* rather than *prevent* subsequent cell necrosis. In dogs, occlusion of a coronary artery for three hours followed by reperfusion results in an infarct the same size as if the occlusion had been permanent (141). In this experiment, the time chosen was three hours because this is the minimal time for estimation of infarct size by staining with tetrazolium salts. Another interpretation of this experimental model is that three hours of ischaemia was sufficient to result in an infarct of maximum size so that reperfusion could not and did not have any beneficial effect. These are difficult arguments to refute but, equally, they are only assertions and not proof that reperfusion damage does not exist.

Proof of the existence of reperfusion damage rests with either of two criteria:
Description of a biochemical sequence of events at the moment of reperfusion which causes myocardial damage; or
Use of an intervention at the moment of reperfusion which reduces infarct size. The latter condition is pivotal.

Numerous pharmacological interventions have been shown to increase recovery of the myocardium after a period of ischaemia, but most need to be introduced before the onset of ischaemia and thus have limited clinical application. Such interventions exert benefit through a cardioplegic effect (reduction of myocardial contraction resulting in a lower rate of consumption of ATP), alteration of coronary flow at the moment of reperfusion, change in systemic haemodynamics to alter oxygen consumption, or alteration of residual flow through the native coronary vessel or collaterals.

These requirements raise important questions for the experimental cardiologist. The measurement of infarct size has a long and somewhat tarnished history. The major difficulty has arisen because of the use of the dog as the experimental animal. Three key points have now emerged:

1. Experiments in dogs attempting to measure infarct size must be blinded and randomized.

2. Consideration must be given to the possibility that observed differences relate to differences in collateral blood flow. Comparison of the plot of area of infarct divided by the area at risk against collateral flow in the presence of intervention and placebo is useful *(125)*.

3. A distinction should be made between infarct size and recovery of contractile function. Usually, but not necessarily, these occur together and are related, but recovery of full contractile function may take several hours or even days (stunned myocardium) *(70)*. However, the area of infarction can also take time to develop. Thus it can be argued that infarct size should be measured approximately 48 hours after

reperfusion following, say, 45 minutes of ischaemia. However, other evidence suggests that, during such a period of time, there is considerable remodelling of the myocardium and infarct expansion. If the experimentalist delays too long, remodelling renders the measurement of infarct size impossible but, if the measurement is made too early, it may underestimate the true size and spuriously suggest a reduction of infarct size when it is merely a delay in the development towards the ultimate infarct size.

Several experiments using agents introduced at the moment of reperfusion provide evidence of reperfusion damage. In the dog, the infusion of superoxide dismutase and catalase at the moment of reperfusion results in a reduction of infarct size (142). The effect appears to be independent of other factors, such as systemic haemodynamics and coronary flow, although these are notoriously difficult to measure and hold constant in the canine model.

In other models, superoxide dismutase increases coronary flow on reperfusion (143,144). Others have used adenosine (145) or fluorocarbons (146) and shown a reduction of infarct size. An important observation is the reduction of infarct size in species other than the dog, such as the rabbit, in which collateral flow is minimal. The most convincing evidence comes from experiments where the calcium concentration in the perfusate is manipulated at the time of reperfusion. Increased recovery of mechanical function has been reported in the working rat heart preparation (147), and improvement in both functional and biochemical parameters in the arterially perfused septum of the rabbit (148,149).

Experiments in single cells (150) show a reoxygenation effect that is difficult to explain unless reoxygenation damage is a real entity. The weakness of these experiments is that they measured myocardial function and not infarct size. Nevertheless, when taken together, they appear to suggest that reperfusion damage is a real phenomenon due to events affecting the myocyte at the moment of reperfusion.

Recently, two pieces of evidence have suggested that reperfusion damage can occur in man. The pattern of the release of enzymes in the coronary sinus following successful thrombolysis is similar (151) to previous observations in isolated tissues. The death rate in the GISSI study of the benefit of thrombolysis was higher during the first 24 hours in those treated with streptokinase (152). This clinical observation is compatible with an early harmful effect of such treatment.

Table 3.8   Possible causes of myocardial damage during ischaemia and on reperfusion

Lack of energy (ATP)

Calcium accumulation and loss of calcium homeostasis

Mechanical stress: Stretching of cells and osmotic pressure

Lipid changes in cell membrane

Sodium/hydrogen/calcium exchange

Free radicals

Table 3.9   Reperfusion damage: Determining factors

Period of ischaemia
  Duration;
  Residual blood flow;
  Myocardial oxygen consumption

Blood flow
  Sudden or slow restoration;
  Endothelial cell damage;
  No reflow phenomenon

Constituents of blood
  Calcium;
  Other ions;
  Temperature

Inflammatory response
  White cells

Intramyocardial haemorrhage

Causes of reperfusion damage

Many hypotheses have been put forward to account for damage on reperfusion and these have been reviewed *(71, 153-155)* (Table 3.8). In addition to the causes of reperfusion damage, there are many factors which determine the severity of the damage (Table 3.9).

Reperfusion is accompanied by a variety of well characterized phenomena (see Table 3.7). If reperfusion occurs early during ischaemia, full recovery results but, after approximately 30 minutes of total global ischaemia, complete functional recovery of the heart muscle does not occur. A similar phenomenon occurs on reoxygenation of the myocardium after a period of hypoxia *(140)*. This has been called the 'oxygen paradox' and the phenomenon 'reoxygenation damage'. There are similarities with another situation, namely, the restoration of normal calcium levels in the perfusate after a period of low calcium perfusion – the 'calcium paradox'. After a period of ischaemia, the phrase 'reperfusion damage' has been used.

> A truism which needs emphasizing is that myocardium inevitably necroses if blood flow is not restored. The phrase 'reperfusion damage' is therefore misleading as, without reperfusion, cell necrosis is inevitable.

Reperfusion is always beneficial in terms of potential recovery of heart muscle. The causes of cell death in reperfused myocardium are a matter of considerable controversy *(71,155)* and a number of hypotheses abound at present (see Table 3.8).

Energy deficiency. Although this is an appealing hypotheses, it is difficult to link cell necrosis with a lack of energy in the form of high-energy phosphates (CP and ATP) *(156)*. Many experiments have shown that the degree of necrosis correlates well with the decrease in high-energy phosphates. Such a correlation would be found between any variable that declined or increased during ischaemia as recovery is linked closely to the duration of ischaemia.

> In order to demonstrate a causal relationship, a mechanism must be identified and shown to be the critical event. Recovery of the ischaemic myocardium can be improved without alteration of the high-energy phosphates. In many tissues, although the high-energy phosphates reach very low levels, the tissue recovers. Thus, ATP consumption, while undoubtedly necessary for recovery, does not appear to be a key requirement.

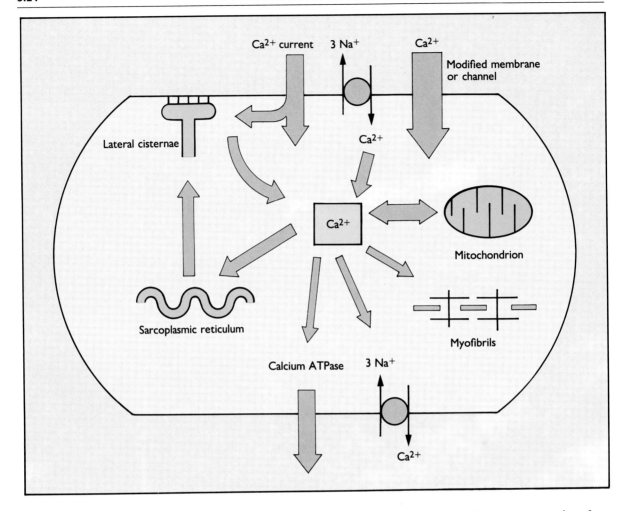

Figure 3.7 Diagrammatic representation of calcium in the myocardium. Calcium enters the cell as the slow calcium current, which increases the cytosolic calcium, leading to contraction, and also causes further release of calcium from the lateral cisternae of the sarcoplasmic reticulum. Cytosolic calcium is lowered by limiting calcium release and by uptake of calcium by the sarcoplasmic reticulum. A net gain of calcium in the normal cell is prevented by mechanisms for the extrusion of calcium. In ischaemia, it appears that the increased calcium influx is through a modified calcium channel or increased permeability of the cell membrane.

Calcium hypothesis. The most popular theory accounting for reperfusion damage is the calcium hypothesis, which states that the sudden influx of calcium on reperfusion is the cause of subsequent cell death (Table 3.10). Calcium homeostasis is a necessary condition for many cellular functions (Figure 3.7). A large gradient is present between the intra- and extracellular fluid and the cell has several systems to maintain the gradient. In the heart, cytosolic calcium is carefully controlled and calcium is a key ion for normal contracture, many enzyme reactions *(157)*, the generation of ATP by the mitochondria *(158)*, membrane stability *(117, 118)* and ion homeostasis. Minor degrees of calcium overload can occur on total recovery and in the absence of cell necrosis *(159)*.

On reperfusion after a period of ischaemia, calcium crosses the cell membrane from the extracellular space and is taken up into the mitochondria where it can be seen as small dark opacities on electron microscopy. When the mitochondria become overloaded with calcium, they are no longer able to generate ATP normally *(158,160)*. Calcium accumulates immediately in the reperfused myocardium *(161-164)*. The net gain is due to an increase of influx and not a reduction of efflux, and

Table 3.10 Final common pathways for reperfusion damage

Loss of ionic homeostasis
→ Calcium accumulation

Membrane damage

Calcium affects:

Mitochondrial function;

Cell membrane stability;

Enzymes;

Sarcoplasmic reticulum;

Myofibrillar contraction

the degree of cell damage relates to the total tissue calcium. Calcium influx occurs in the absence of gross disruption of the cell membrane (see below) and is not inhibited directly by calcium antagonists *(163)*, high extracellular potassium *(163)*, quiescence *(163)* or alpha-blockade *(165)*. It can be inhibited by nickel ions *(153)* and is mimicked by hydrogen or cumene peroxide, but not lysophosphatidylcholine *(165)*. These observations support the idea that calcium influx is at least in part due to modification of the cell membrane at the moment of reoxygenation or reperfusion which results in a massive influx of calcium. This modification may not be to the lipid in the cell membrane, but a more subtle damage to the receptor itself so that the channel loses its ability to prevent calcium moving down the concentration gradient.

The essential question is what is it that brings about the increased influx of calcium, and is the influx a consequence of damage to the cell membrane and movement of calcium down its concentration gradient (extracellular calcium 10^{-3} M, intracellular calcium 10^{-6} M) or is it a result of the normal function of physiological ion control mechanisms in the presence of pathological ionic gradients?

The influx of calcium has been extensively described on both reperfusion *(161-164)* and reoxygenation *(153,166)*. Although there are many biochemical differences between these two events, the alteration of calcium exchange in each appears to be almost identical. Both reoxygenation and reperfusion result in a release of enzymes, calcium influx and failure to recover complete mechanical function.

The unidirectional fluxes of calcium and the net changes in the tissue have been well described. In order to understand further the relation of damage to alterations of calcium homeostasis, it is necessary to obtain information on the concentration of calcium in the cell during reperfusion (Table 3.11; *119-123*). Experiments have also been reported in hypoxia and during reoxygenation *(79,167,168)* where it has been argued that the damage to the cell on reoxygenation precedes the rise of cytosolic calcium *(169)*; others have reported the opposite result, making this a controversial point. The difficulties in interpreting the results of these numerous experiments are due to the variation in experimental models and major problems with the use of different methods for the measurement of cytosolic calcium concentration; for example, 5FBAPTA can only be used when the cell membrane and cell organelles are intact. The signal from aequorin is sensitive to magnesium and it is now known that the increase in cytosolic magnesium concen-

Table 3.11   Cytosolic calcium in ischaemia

Author	Date	Species	Indicator	Time	Systolic	Diastolic
Steenbergen et al.	1987	Rat	5FBAPTA	6–15 min	–	+ (at 10 min)
Marban et al.	1987	Ferret	5FBAPTA	10–20 min	–	+ (×3 at 6 min)
Allen et al.	1989	Ferret	Aequorin	10 min	+	0
Lee et al.	1987	Rabbit	Indo+1	90 s	+	+
				3 min	0	0

tration is at least fivefold in the first 15 minutes of ischaemia *(97)*. Some indicators, such as indo-1, may be selectively concentrated in endothelial cells, thus partly invalidating the conclusions drawn. Lack of knowledge concerning the cytosolic calcium concentration is still the greatest obstacle towards understanding the role of calcium homeostasis in ischaemia.

Mechanical and osmotic stress. Some authors have argued that, at the time of reperfusion, there is an increased contracture of the myocardial cells and that this force pulls adjacent cells apart, thus disrupting the cell membrane at the intercalated discs where a cell is joined to its neighbours *(170)*. Alternatively, changes of osmotic pressure on reperfusion may cause the cell to be disrupted and calcium to flow into the cell down its concentration gradient *(171,172)*. The disruption of the cell membrane is said to cause the inward movement of calcium and destruction of ionic gradients which are essential to cell survival. However, there are experimental conditions in which the rise in resting tension is either absent or very small and yet recovery does not occur *(153)*. The cell membrane would need to have been weakened by other biochemical events during ischaemia as the healthy myocyte is resistant to substantial changes of osmotic pressure.

Both of these mechanisms require major disruption of the cell membrane to have occurred. Although they may contribute to the development of cell necrosis, they are unlikely to be of central importance. Calcium influx can occur without extracellular markers gaining access to the intracellular space *(153,173)*, and is inhibited by a small ion such as nickel. Intracellular potassium ions are not released into the extracellular fluid at the moment of reoxygenation *(174)*. Total destruction of the cell membrane is a late event and not a determining factor in the development of necrosis.

Lipid changes in membranes. Alterations of the lipid structure have been described and lead to the formation of blebs and loss of enzyme *(117,118)*. The function of the cell membrane and channels within it may be affected by the activation of lipases during ischaemia and by the accumulation of lipid moieties such as acyl-CoA and lysophospholipids. Recently, it has been shown that sarcolemmal vesicles are sensitized to the effects of oxygen radicals by lipases *(175)*. Measurements in the intact heart indicate that such changes occur very late in ischaemia, long after the time at which reperfusion leads to no recovery whatsoever *(124)*.

Sodium-calcium exchange. The hypothesis has been proposed that sodium-hydrogen exchange is inhibited during ischaemia by the low extracellular pH *(176)*. On reperfusion, hydrogen ions move out of the cell in exchange for sodium. The increase in the intracellular sodium concentration activates sodium-calcium exchange. The overall consequence is an increased calcium influx due to a net exchange of hydrogen and calcium ions. This hypothesis in its simplest form is unlikely to be correct as calcium influx occurs on reoxygenation and reperfusion and, during hypoxia, the extracellular pH is not greatly altered. Nevertheless, it is conceivable that sodium-calcium exchange is a relevant mechanism and requires other factors to initiate this series of ionic events.

Alteration of extracellular sodium does influence the survival of ischaemic myocardium *(177,178)*, but the direct demonstration of sodium-calcium exchange is lacking *(179,180)*.

The essential information for any hypothesis seeking to explain reperfusion damage is the cytosolic concentration of sodium, hydrogen and calcium ions. Evidence is scanty and conflicting.

Isolated myocytes can 'round up' in the absence of an increase of cytosolic calcium *(169)*. Early in hypoxia, cytosolic calcium does not increase, but may do so when contracture develops *(168)*. Information on sodium is also sparse. During the first 15 minutes of ischaemia, cytosolic sodium may not increase *(112)* because a reduced influx allows the functional, but less active, sodium pump to resist any change *(181)*. During hypoxia, most *(79,179,181-183)*, but not all *(184)*, reports indicate a substantial increase of cytosolic sodium particularly when the severity of hypoxia is sufficient to cause a rise in resting tension. A problem then arises in accounting for the lack of an increased calcium during hypoxia rather than on reoxygenation.

A possible explanation is that the cytosolic calcium does increase during hypoxia, but a large increase of total tissue calcium is not observed because the uptake of calcium into the mitochondria is inhibited by other metabolites and the lack of oxygen. There are major technical difficulties with the currently available methods of measuring cytosolic ion concentrations under pathological conditions. Ion-selective electrodes may provide values from unrepresentative cells, and techniques using calcium markers require an intact cell membrane.

Radicals. Currently, the most fashionable idea for the cause of reperfusion damage is that it is the function of the cell membrane by oxygen or other radicals generated at the moment of reperfusion *(76)*. Free radicals are a chemical species with an unpaired electron. They participate in many chemical reactions and are generated from many sources in different cell types (Figure 3.8; Table 3.12). The best described radicals are those associated with oxygen, but other moieties, such as lipids, can also form radicals.

This hypothesis is attractive because it would account for the similarity between the events occurring on reoxygenation of the myocardium with those observed on reperfusion. Calcium influx can be mimicked by peroxides *(165)*. During ischaemia, the enzyme systems used by the cell to protect itself from radicals have a reduced activity *(185)*, and there is evidence of an increased production of radicals *(186-188)*.

Much of the evidence for this hypothesis, however, has rested on experiments using inhibitors of questionable specificity and affecting only one mechanism of radical production

Figure 3.8 Some well described reactions involving free radicals.

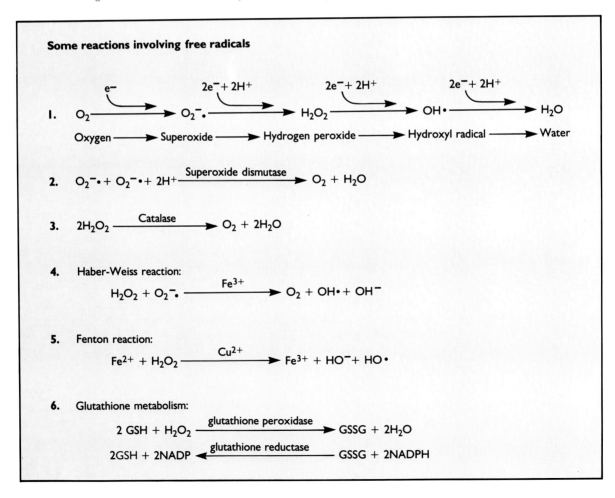

Some reactions involving free radicals

1. $O_2 \xrightarrow{e^-} O_2^- \cdot \xrightarrow{2e^- + 2H^+} H_2O_2 \xrightarrow{2e^- + 2H^+} OH \cdot \xrightarrow{2e^- + 2H^+} H_2O$

   Oxygen ⟶ Superoxide ⟶ Hydrogen peroxide ⟶ Hydroxyl radical ⟶ Water

2. $O_2^- \cdot + O_2^- \cdot + 2H^+ \xrightarrow{\text{Superoxide dismutase}} O_2 + H_2O$

3. $2H_2O_2 \xrightarrow{\text{Catalase}} O_2 + 2H_2O$

4. Haber-Weiss reaction:

   $H_2O_2 + O_2^- \cdot \xrightarrow{Fe^{3+}} O_2 + OH \cdot + OH^-$

5. Fenton reaction:

   $Fe^{2+} + H_2O_2 \xrightarrow{Cu^{2+}} Fe^{3+} + HO^- + HO \cdot$

6. Glutathione metabolism:

   $2\,GSH + H_2O_2 \xrightarrow{\text{glutathione peroxidase}} GSSG + 2H_2O$

   $2GSH + 2NADP \xleftarrow{\text{glutathione reductase}} GSSG + 2NADPH$

(116,187,188). Radicals may be generated from white cells, from catecholamines in the endothelium, in the cell membrane or in mitochondria. Removal of white cells has been suggested to reduce infarct size *(189)*, but they are absent from many preparations in which reperfusion damage has been demonstrated. Allopurinol may also have a beneficial effect on infarct size *(187)* because it inhibits xanthine oxidase, which may contribute to radical formation by an interaction between hypoxanthine and oxygen. However, not all experiments with allopurinol or radical scavengers have shown a reduction in infarct size *(187,188,190)*. The enzyme xanthine oxidase is apparently absent in the rabbit and present in only small amounts in man.

Several studies have shown a beneficial effect with the addition of superoxide dismutase *(188)* to the perfusate or blood before reperfusion *(142,144)*. This substance can alter coronary blood flow *(143,144)*. Thus, not all of its effects are necessarily due to the destruction of radicals. The enzyme may not cross the cell membrane and it may be that, in some models where no effect of superoxide dismutase has been observed, radicals are formed in mitochondria or in the inner surface of the cell membrane and are therefore inaccessible to the enzyme.

Reversal of reperfusion damage

Many interventions known to reduce the effects of ischaemia, such as hypothermia, cardioplegia or the calcium antagonists, are generally only effective if applied to the myocardium prior to the period of ischaemia. They have no benefit if they are applied at the time of reperfusion. Recently, some interventions, particularly a lowering of the extracellular calcium concentration *(147,148)* and introduction of oxygen scavengers *(142)*, adenosine *(145)* or fluorocarbons *(146)*, have led to an improved recovery of the myocardium. These experiments appear to suggest that some of the events occurring at the moment of reperfusion are damaging to the myocardium and alteration of these events can lead to greater recovery of the muscle. An important question, however, is whether this increased recovery of the muscle is only a hastening of recovery which would have occurred if the muscle had been reperfused for a prolonged period of time. At present, this proposition is apparently unlikely to be correct.

Reperfusion of ischaemic myocardial tissue is limited by a decrease in the maximum capacity for vasodilatation. The biochemical events at the moment of reperfusion do not appear to be merely the manifestation of previous ischaemia, nor are they the markers of inevitable cell death.

Table 3.12 Radicals and reperfusion damage

Nature
Superoxide, hydrogen peroxide, hydroxyl, organic

Site of origin
Blood
Catecholamines, white cells
Endothelial cell
Xanthine
Myocardial cell
Mitochondria, membranes

Site of action
Endothial cell
Myocardial cell
Lipids in cell membrane
Membrane proteins

Reperfusion damage is a real phenomenon which can be modified, although the underlying mechanisms and their relative importance are still not understood. It is possible that no single cause will be found, but that the phenomenon has a multifactorial origin. Nevertheless, experimental work does indicate that reperfusion damage can be circumvented, providing optimism for the pharmacologist. Drug therapy aimed at the prevention of reperfusion damage could logically be combined with thrombolytic therapy in the treatment of acute myocardial infarction in man.

Preconditioning of the ischaemic myocardium
Acute myocardial infarction in man is not usually associated with sudden and complete occlusion of a coronary artery but, rather, increasingly frequent episodes of transient ischaemia *(129,130)*. Thus, most animal models of ischaemia are not comparable to myocardial infarction in man. Breakdown of an atheromatous plaque and platelet aggregation on the exposed surface of the vessel wall is the probable cause of many myocardial infarcts *(74,75)* (Table 3.13). A thrombus is formed and complex biochemical interactions initiated *(191,192)*. In those who develop infarcts with Q-waves *(193)* on ECG, thrombosis is a common occurrence after one hour from the onset of chest pain and decreases in frequency in the subsequent few hours as a result of spontaneous thrombolysis. In patients with non-Q-wave infarction *(194)*, thrombosis is not common early after the onset of pain, but increases in frequency over the following eight hours. These observations show that, in man, the onset of ischaemia is not sudden. Abrupt occlusion of a coronary artery in a dog is a poor model of infarction in man.

In the last few years, numerous studies of repetitive coronary occlusions have been reported. Short periods of ischaemia have been shown to cause mechanical changes lasting weeks *(195,196)*. The loss of adenine nucleotides is not replaced for several days *(23)*. The loss of functional capacity has been attributed to modification of excitation-contraction coupling rather than energy availability *(198)* ('stunned myocardium'; see below). Even five minutes of ischaemia results in functional changes for more than three hours *(199)*.

The effect of repeated coronary occlusion is paradoxical. In Langendorff perfused rats *(200)* and anaesthetized dogs *(201)*, exposure to a period of hypoxia or four to five minute periods of ischaemia reduced infarct size and increased recovery of mechanical function during a subsequent period of more prolonged ischaemia.

Table 3.13 Total coronary occlusion in myocardial infarction

Q-wave infarction		Non-Q-wave infarction	
Hours after symptoms	Occluded (%)	Hours after symptoms	Occluded (%)
0–4	87	0–24	26
4–6	85	24–72	37
6–12	68	72–7 days	42
12–24	65		

DeWood et al., N Engl J Med, 1980; **303**: 897-902
1986; **315**: 417-423

The mechanism is probably not related to ATP concentration in the tissue *(200)* nor is it due to the opening or development of collaterals delivering more blood to the myocardium. Metabolic products may reduce the strength of contraction so that the accumulation of damaging products is diminished during the more prolonged period of ischaemia *(198)*. The nature of the relevant metabolic products is unknown. Lactate, hydrogen ions and NADH have been suggested, although myocardium can be exposed to high concentrations of lactate without any harmful results. Alternatively, the phenomenon of preconditioning may be due to glycogen depletion, improved flux in the glycosylation pathway, altered contraction, a reduced demand for ATP, an effect on collagen and the structure of the myocardial lattice or the function of the sarcoplasmic reticulum. More subtle effects on ionic channels are another possibility.

Stunned and hibernating heart muscle
Although after short periods of ischaemia the partial recovery of the function of the heart is rapid, careful measurements have shown that further recovery occurs over days and even weeks *(195,196)*. Despite restoration of flow and the absence of ischaemia, the consequences of ischaemia to the myocardium can last for hours and even weeks.

Cardiac function can remain depressed after periods of ischaemia for up to four weeks. If function is depressed in the presence of normal coronary flow and with absence of necrosis, the myocardium is said to be 'stunned' *(70)*. If function is reduced in the presence of continuing reduction of blood flow, but necrosis does not immediately result, the myocardium is said to be 'hibernating' *(202)*.

The difference between these two entities is somewhat arbitrary, and the mechanism(s) is uncertain. One proposal is that, during ischaemia, high-energy phosphates are broken down to xanthine and hypoxanthine and these moieties are lost from the myocardium. The normal energy state of the myocardium is not restored until these high-energy phosphates have been resynthesized, a process which may take up to a week. There is evidence both for and against this hypothesis *(203,204)*. The loss of potassium, which is known to occur during short periods of ischaemia, is not restored for up to 30 minutes; repeated episodes of ischaemia may therefore lead to an accumulated loss of ions from the heart. The contractile function of the stunned myocardium can be restored by the infusion of inotropic agents or an increase in the extracellular calcium concentration, suggesting that the abnormality is unrelated to the contractile proteins.

There is some evidence suggesting that the abnormality is due to the effect of oxygen radicals, as the effect can be inhibited by interventions which reduce radical accumulation. Others have argued that the effect is a consequence of damage to the extracellular matrix of the myocardium. This author at present believes that stunned, hibernating and preconditioned myocardium may all be interrelated as manifestations of damage to the function of ionic channels in the myocardium, in particular, calcium channels in the sarcoplasmic reticulum.

Determinants of infarct size

In the 1970s, the belief was that a myocardial infarct was surrounded by myocardium which had a marginal blood flow and could be regarded as 'jeopardized' or 'threatened'. Experiments were undertaken with a variety of drugs and interventions which appeared to indicate that 'infarct' size could be reduced *(91)*. Subsequently, clinical trials were undertaken with various drugs and, certainly in the case of beta-blockers, it has been shown that, when used in patients after myocardial infarction, there is a reduction in subsequent death and reinfarction *(6)*. The original experiments in animals and isolated tissue that demonstrated the supposed reduction of infarct size have been challenged *(13)*. The challenge has been based largely on the question of whether the experiments showed a reduction of infarct size or merely a delay in the development of the infarct. The issue is complicated by criticism of the techniques used to demonstrate the amount of muscle at risk of infarcting on vessel occlusion and the true final size of an infarct. Furthermore, there is the important question of whether animals that die during an experiment are excluded from the final analysis of results. If this is the case and those animals had the larger infarcts, then only animals with smaller infarcts have survived and an apparent reduction of infarct size is observed. More recent experiments have not confirmed early enthusiasm and, indeed, there is now strong evidence indicating that the whole concept of infarct size reduction is flawed.

There are wide species variations in anatomical arrangement of the coronary arteries (126). The guinea-pig has such an extensive collateral flow that it is almost impossible to induce an infarct by occlusion of a coronary artery. In the pig, most of the coronary arteries are end-arteries. The dog has extensive collateral circulation within the endocardium. Man, in general, appears to have end-arteries in his coronary system but, in the presence of coronary artery disease, collaterals develop over the years, producing an anatomy somewhat similar to that in the dog. These observations are essential for interpretation of animal data. In the pig (without collaterals) and the dog (no collateral circulation in the epicardium), occlusion of a coronary artery leads to a clearly demarcated infarct on the endocardial surface of the heart. With time, the infarct spreads from the endocardial to the epicardial surface, producing a full-thickness infarct (13,205). The edge of the infarct does not alter. Why the endocardium is apparently more vulnerable than the epicardium is not clear, but may relate to a different wall tension, metabolic rate or distribution of blood vessels. Necrosis begins in the subendocardium independent of collateral flow and wall tension (206).

Detailed investigation of the nature of the infarct edge shows that there is no border zone (207) (or it is less than one cell in thickness) and that the capillary beds supplied by the normal tissue interdigitate or are immediately adjacent.

These observations have an important clinical significance as it is unlikely that infarct size can be altered except by restoration of coronary blood flow. Blood flow may be increased by opening of preexisting collaterals, by development of new collaterals (a process requiring a minimum of 48 hours) or by redistribution of the collateral flow between the epicardium and endocardium.

An important issue is the use of myocardial enzyme release to measure the size of an infarct. Simple consideration of this method suggests that it is erroneous. In a severe infarct, there is little blood flow to the centre of the infarct and the enzymes are not reduced from that area of muscle whereas, in a small infarct, a small residual coronary flow is present and the enzymes are released. Thus, the amount of enzyme released is not truly related to the size of the infarct. A further problem arises on consideration of the mechanism by which enzyme is released from cells *(208)*. If the cell membrane is disrupted, enzymes pass out of the myocardial cell, but it is also clear that, in early ischaemia and on reperfusion after short periods of ischaemia, enzymes can pass out of the myocardial cell without gross disruption of the cell membrane. Thus, small increases in blood enzymes in the presence of chest pain are not necessarily an indication of cell necrosis.

The determinants of infarct size (Table 3.14) are the duration of ischaemia, anatomy of the occluded coronary bed, presence and extent of collaterals, and rate of oxygen consumption at the onset of ischaemia. Recent experiments to assess these factors, in which animals were randomized and the experimentalist blinded, have failed to confirm earlier studies claiming that drugs such as beta-blockers *(1)* and calcium antagonists *(125)* can reduce infarct size either after permanent occlusion or occlusion for three hours.

Myocardial ischaemia in man
Angina pectoris and angioplasty

A major challenge in cardiology is to understand the precise cause of the symptom, angina pectoris. The presence of angina is poor evidence of the presence of ischaemia; as much as 25% of all myocardial infarctions may be silent *(209)*, and numerous episodes of myocardial ischaemia are not associated with chest pain *(210,211)*. As pain is a late manifestation (60 seconds) of myocardial ischaemia, it may be that the initiating factor for pain is the rise in extracellular potassium concentration. When a threshold is reached, sufficient nerve fibres may be activated to give rise to the sensations that clinicians call 'angina'. The perception of pain by the patient is variable, depending on the pain threshold. Angina was initially used to describe a feeling of tightness in the throat and lower neck. Part of this symptom may occur because of a rise in the left atrial pressure associated with a reduction in cardiac contraction. The sensation in the chest would then have some features in common with acute heart failure.

Angina pectoris is a characteristic pain in the chest usually indicating heart disease. Indeed, some physicians now use the term angina to describe only chest pain arising from the heart. Such use assumes the cause of the symptom before it has been established. This is not the original meaning of angina pectoris and is not the sense in which the word is used by the present author.

Table 3.14   Determinants of myocardial infarct size

Duration of ischaemic episode

Anatomical distribution of occluded artery

Presence and extent of existing collaterals

Residual flow through native vessels ('stuttering ischaemia')

Oxygen consumption at moment of occlusion

The most common cause of angina in the Western world is obstruction of the coronary arteries by atheroma. The diagnosis carries important consequences with regard to treatment and prognosis. The best predictor of a coronary event (angina, myocardial infarction or sudden death) is the previous demonstration of atheromatous coronary artery disease. The clinical skills of physicians are finely honed towards making this diagnosis and their view of other conditions, which may mimic the symptoms of atheromatous coronary artery disease, is conditioned by experience with this common entity.

> Angina can be due to myocardial ischaemia, which may be caused not by a limitation of coronary blood flow but by other mechanisms, such as increased work of the heart (as in aortic stenosis), altered oxygen levels in the blood or rheological abnormalities of the blood. All of these diseases can be manifest as ischaemia of the myocardium.

All of the above presumes that angina is due to either an increased consumption of oxygen or an increased workload imposed upon the heart. A further consideration is that coronary flow can be altered by factors which change during exercise or by the circumstances which precipitated the angina. Coronary flow can be altered by changes in either resistance or perfusion pressure (Table 3.15). Many factors besides a fixed obstruction or contraction of the smooth muscle (dynamic stenosis) can alter resistance. Likewise, the determinants of perfusion pressure throughout the myocardium are many and complex.

Angina pectoris is not easily diagnosed from a clinical history alone. Many entities have been described over the years to account for the presence of angina-like chest pain in cases where the physician has remained unconvinced that the mechanism was 'true' myocardial ischaemia or that the pain was arising from the heart. Thus, terms such as 'Da Costa's syndrome' *(212)*, 'effort syndrome' *(212)*, 'neurocirculatory aesthesia', 'anxiety neurosis', 'vasoregulatory aesthesia', 'soldier's irritable heart' *(213)* and 'hyperventilation syndrome' have been used. Furthermore, pain genuinely arising from the oesophagus, musculoskeletal structures or of a psychological origin may masquerade as angina. The clinical diagnosis of angina pectoris arising from the heart is difficult and physicians are frequently mistaken.

The recent introduction of angioplasty has provided a model whereby the early effects of ischaemia can be studied in man. It is apparent that the monophasic action potential shortens after approximately the sixteenth heart beat *(90)* and as contraction falls *(82)*, potassium is lost from the myocardium *(109)*

Table 3.15   Causes of changing coronary flow

Resistance
Physiological vasoconstriction
Pathological vasoconstriction
  Localizing factor
  Trigger factor
Passive changes
Intravascular plugging
Compression by extravascular (muscle) forces

Perfusion pressure
Blood pressure
Pressure in coronary sinus
Transmural pressures
Wall tension

and intracellular acidosis develops *(68)*. Thus, angioplasty has provided evidence that many of the phenomena known to occur in animals also occur in man.

Mechanism of myocardial infarction

Although the symptoms and clinical picture of myocardial infarction had been described earlier, it was not until 1910 *(214,215)* that the entity was clearly described. The cause of myocardial infarction has long been the subject of a debate centred on whether thrombosis in a coronary artery occurred prior to and was the cause of the infarction or occurred subsequent to the infarction and was therefore a consequence.

> Recent evidence and popular opinion strongly favours the view that thrombosis occurs prior to infarction and is a causal mechanism, but this view may be overstated *(83,84)*.

Myocardial infarction has no single cause. If causes such as emboli are put aside, the central issue is the origin of the myocardial infarction in the presence of coronary artery disease. According to the most popular scheme, there is a rupture and/or haemorrhage into an atheromatous plaque. Collagen in the wall of the artery is brought, into contact with the bloodstream, allowing platelets *(38)* to adhere to the collagen and eventually to aggregate, become activated and form a thrombus which finally occludes the coronary artery; infarction of the myocardial tissue supplied by the artery ensues. Vasoconstriction of the coronary artery may occur, if it is anatomically possible, as a result of the release of vasoconstricting substances (ADP, ATP, 5-hydroxytryptamine, thromboxane A_2) by the platelets in the developing thrombus. These substances may normally be vasodilators because they stimulate the release of EDRF, but cause vasoconstriction in the absence of endothelium.

There are other causes of a variable obstruction in a coronary artery, but the key evidence in favour of this hypothesis is that unstable atheromatous plaques are common findings in patients dying with coronary artery disease *(24,74,75)*, and total occlusion of coronary arteries has been demonstrated in more than 70% of patients between one and four hours after the onset of chest pain *(193,194)*. After that time, the incidence of coronary occlusion declines, presumably due to spontaneous dissolution of the thrombus by natural thrombolytic mechanisms.

However, examination of coronary arteries between one and four hours after the onset of chest pain does not resolve the problem of whether thrombosis occurs before or after the development of myocardial infarction. This evidence merely focuses interest on the first hour after the onset of chest pain. It is possible and even probable that unstable plaques are a rare event in individual patients with coronary artery disease, but because many subjects have coronary artery disease, they occur relatively frequently. Not all unstable plaques lead to myocardial infarction. It is possible that myocardial infarction itself causes splinting and other changes in the coronary artery which contribute to the development of so-called plaque rupture. Data on the incidence of thrombosis from studies of patients in sudden death are conflicting and do not contribute greatly to the debate as the causes of sudden death may differ substantially from the causes of acute myocardial infarction *(216)*.

There may be different causes in different populations. There are several alternative hypotheses for the origin of myocardial infarction, including platelet emboli, vasoconstriction and compression of the myocardial capillaries by contracture developing in the myocardial muscle *(217)*. In the author's opinion, the hypothesis that myocardial infarction is due to thrombosis in the coronary artery is overly simplistic and is accepted too dogmatically at present.

The mechanism of myocardial infarction is likely to be multifactorial and the contribution of each factor possibly varies from one individual to another. Important considerations appear to be:

Severity of coronary stenosis;

Ability of platelets to adhere to the wall of the atheromatous plaque (rupture);

Contraction of the smooth muscle in the wall of the artery;

Preexisting anatomy of the atheromatous plaque allowing shortening of the smooth muscle;

Presence of collaterals;

Degree of activity of the natural thrombolytic system;

Degree of compression of capillaries in the distal coronary bed by contracting myocardium.

Several studies *(219)* have now shown that coronary events such as anginal episodes, ST-segment depression on ECG, sudden death and myocardial infarction, occur more frequently in the early hours of the morning between six o'clock and midday. Many physiological processes have a similar circadian rhythm and some, such as the factors involved in the thrombotic process, may be related to the occurrence of infarction. The most easily understood theory is that the increased workload associated with waking up in the morning provides sufficient stimulation to alter the balance of factors, thus allowing rupture of an atheromatous plaque to result in total occlusion rather than spontaneous healing. The circadian rhythm of cardiac events is not large and cardiac events arise at all times of day and night. In addition, the nature of the infarct, treatment with drugs, cigarette-smoking and diabetes may override a circadian rhythm (219). There is, therefore, no clinical application of this phenomenon in, for example, the timing of the provision of resources.

Whatever the mechanism of infarction, the consequences are well described. In some patients, there is expansion of the myocardium over the subsequent days (Figure 3.9). Much recent interest has been concerned with the nature of this expansion and how cell slippage comes about. The extracellular matrix must be damaged in order to allow cells to slip and realign. White cells accumulate in the infarcted myocardium within 30 minutes and may be a key factor in determining the pattern of the repair process.

Animal models of infarction have shown that the fall of the ejection fraction in medium-sized myocardial infarctions may be prevented by treatment at the time of the infarction with angiotensin-converting enzyme (ACE) inhibitors. Studies in man have shown less clear results. One study failed to show any significant differences between the treated and placebo groups except in a selected subgroup of patients with anterior myocardial infarction. This hypothesis needs further investigation. A second study (Fig. 10. *See p. 3.48*) has shown a small effect with an ACE inhibitor, but it is not certain that the effect was a consequence of the presence of the drug or whether remodelling of the myocardium had occurred which would have persisted without the presence of the drug.

Figure 3.9 Following acute myocardial infarction, there is remodelling of the ventricles which, in some patients, may be considerable. Enlargement of the ventricle may be due to changes in both the ischaemic and non-ischaemic tissues. From Eaton, *N Engl J Med* 1979; **300**: 57.

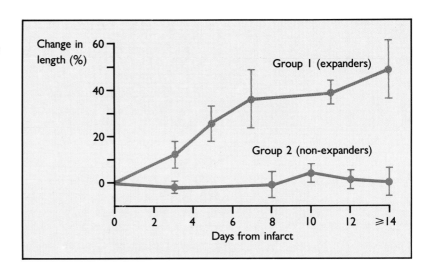

Neurohumoral activation occurs in myocardial infarction and is similar to the activation found in mild heart failure. Whether inhibition of the renin-angiotensin system is advantageous is still not known nor is it clear whether the possible advantages of ACE inhibition result immediately after infarction or can be manifest if the drug is given some time later. ACE inhibitors may exert advantageous effects on the ischaemic myocardium itself, and may favourably alter the haemodynamics or affect the processes involved in repair of the myocardium and hypertrophy. There are potential dangers in early use of ACE inhibitors, in particular, the acute lowering of perfusion pressure.

Stuttering ischaemia

If myocardial infarction is caused by the sudden and total occlusion of a coronary artery, in the absence of collateral flow, the myocardium will then survive for only approximately 40 minutes. It is unlikely that interventions can be applied within this time. However, if the occlusion is not sudden or if there is a collateral blood flow supplying a limited quantity of blood, then the time course over which cell necrosis develops will be greatly extended. Studies of patients very early in the development of infarction indicate that ST segments vary considerably *(129,130)* on surface ECG and may change from moment to moment, so-called stuttering ischaemia. Mechanisms limiting blood flow vary with time in part because of alteration in the degree of smooth muscle vasoconstriction by washout of ions, natural lysis of a thrombus by the normal thrombolytic mechanisms of the body, or alterations of endothelial cell function *(64)*.

If stuttering ischaemia is a reality and common in myocardial infarction, it then becomes an important concept because it greatly lengthens the time available to the physician for introducing an intervention to increase blood flow or to deliver drugs to delay myocardial necrosis until blood flow can be restored.

Stunned myocardium

As indicated above, after an acute myocardial ischaemia, myocardial function and many metabolic changes do not recover immediately but may persist for several weeks. Chest pain has clearly been shown to be a poor indicator of myocardial ischaemia. Patients with angina have frequent episodes of ST-segment changes on surface ECG and only a proportion of these are associated with chest pain *(210,211)*. If coronary arteries are occluded frequently and regularly, it is possible that the myocardium remains 'stunned' almost continuously, giving rise to a reduction in contraction and a picture indistinguishable from the older concept of 'chronic ischaemia'. Repeated episodes of ischaemia may initiate processes leading to myocardial infarction, although the accumulative effect of repeated episodes of ischaemia is contested.

Thrombolysis

The availability of a variety of new thrombolytic agents *(154,191,192)* and recent evidence that thrombosis is an important cause of myocardial infarction have given rise to great interest in the clinical application of these substances *(191, 192)*. Initial results (Table 3.16) appear to indicate that occluded coronary arteries can be opened and that, if patients are treated early, reopening of the coronary artery is accompanied by an improvement of left ventricular function. A recent study (GISSI 2) has shown that the benefits of streptokinase are similar to tissue-plasminogen activator (t-PA). These findings are entirely compatible with the results of earlier animal experiments. However, reocclusion of the coronary artery in man is a problem to be overcome. The expectations of thrombolytic therapy should not be set too high. Only 70% of patients with myocardial infarction have an occluded coronary artery at one hour; of these, only 70% can be opened by thrombolytic therapy, and up to 50% may reocclude within the following days. In a proportion of patients (±40%), the thrombotic processes may not be the key mechanism for the occurrence of myocardial infarction but may be a secondary event. Taking these figures together, thrombolytic therapy would be expected to be of some benefit, but not as a panacea for the treatment of such a complex and multifactorial entity as myocardial infarction.

Thrombolytic therapy is effective in the treatment of myocardial infarction. The greatest benefit is observed in patients who received treatment within one hour of the onset of chest pain *(8)* (Table 3.17).

Two problems face the clinician: First, further treatment, such as coronary artery surgery or angioplasty, may be necessary to prevent reocclusion of the artery in the following week or year.

Second, many patients will not reach medical attention within one hour and, for them, the benefits of thrombolysis are reduced, but are nevertheless present up to approximately eight hours.

The solution is readily apparent, namely, the provision of some form of therapy which delays cell death until thrombolysis can be instituted or becomes effective (Table 3.18).

Table 3.16 Thrombolysis in acute myocardial infarction

Study	Agent	n	0–3/6 hours	3/6–24 hours	Duration of administration (min)
			Mortality reduction (%)		
			Time to onset of pain		
ISIS-2	Streptokinase + aspirin vs placebo	8 592	53%	32–38%	60
AIMS	APSAC + heparin vs placebo + heparin	1 004	47%	–	5
ASSET	rt-PA + heparin vs placebo	? 5 000	24%	–	180
ISAM	Streptokinase vs placebo	1 741	20%	12%	60
GISSI	Streptokinase vs placebo	11 806	23%	6%	60

Such therapy will be given after the onset of severe myocardial ischaemia, when alteration of metabolite production is almost impossible as they have already been formed. A more promising approach is to introduce a drug(s) which would prevent reperfusion damage and limit the extent of eventual necrosis. Diltiazem *(220)* has been tested in such a role despite the disappointing results of trials using calcium antagonists in myocardial infarction. Superoxide dismutase is another agent under investigation.

After the use of thrombolytic drugs and any additional substances, the problems then facing the physician are the timing of further investigations, long-term prevention of atheroma and long-term prevention of recurrent cardiac events.

Table 3.17 GISSI study: Benefit in relation to onset of symptoms

	Streptokinase	Control	Change (%)	p
<1 h	8.2	15.4	−47	0.0001
<3 h	9.2	12.0	−23	0.0005
3–6 h	11.7	14.1	−17	NS
6–9 h	12.6	14.1	−11	NS
9–12 h	15.8	13.6	+16	NS

Lancet 1986; i: 397-401

In the future, drugs may be available which modify the repair process of the myocardium. Recanalization may itself modify the nature of myocardial repair and infarct expansion. If this is true, the effects of thrombolytic therapy will extend beyond the reduction of loss of contractile myocardium.

Q-wave and non-Q-wave infarction

In the past, myocardial infarction has been considered by clinicians to be either full-thickness or partial-thickness infarction. Damage to the myocardium not extending across the whole myocardial wall usually affected the endocardium more than the epicardium (endocardial ischaemia). This distinction was thought to be related to changes on ECG, Q-waves being an indicator of a full-thickness infarct. More recent investigation has shown that this link between ECG findings and pathology is incorrect. At present, myocardial infarction is often classified as either Q-wave or non-Q-wave infarction without reference to the pathology. Difficulties arise with regard to posterior infarcts and prominent R waves in lead V1 and to the importance of ST-segment elevation or depression.

The incidence of non-Q-wave infarction is between 20 and 30% of all infarcts. It is probable that the incidence has increased over the last 20 years, although it is difficult to be sure whether this apparent increase reflects a change in referring and admission policies, a true effect or the consequence of treatment.

The key reason for emphasizing this difference is the belief that full-thickness myocardial infarction is related to total occlusion of a single major coronary vessel. Partial-thickness infarction may have a different pathology. Total occlusion of a single vessel may be followed by early reperfusion. Thus, the wave front of myocardial ischaemia is halted and the only detectable damage is to the endocardium. Alternatively, partial-thickness infarction may reflect the anatomical basis of the lesion(s) leading to thrombosis. Yet another explanation is that the initial pathological mechanism is different. Non-Q-wave infarction may be associated with a greater degree of vasoconstriction and stuttering ischaemia.

A large body of data indicates that non-Q-wave infarction is associated with less damage to the myocardium. Thus, enzyme elevation is less, positive radionuclide scans are fewer, PET (positron emission tomography) scans show greater heterogeneity, thallium scans showing redistribution are more common, and echocardiograms are more likely to be normal. No difference is found in the number of diseased vessels, distribution of plaques, location of the lesion in the infarct-related vessel and amount of myocardium at risk.

Table 3.18 Further immediate objectives with thrombolytic therapy

Prevent reperfusion damage

Maximize blood flow (patency is not reflow)

Modify inflammatory response

Prevent reocclusion

Non-Q-wave infarction is not a benign condition and there is a higher rate of late infarction. The early mortality is less but, in the long-term, the difference in mortality between Q-wave and non-Q-wave infarction is slight. There is the possibility of a higher rate of postinfarction angina in non-Q-wave infarction, but that is under dispute. There is also controversy over the possibility that those with non-Q-wave infarction have a more developed collateral circulation so that, at the time of vessel occlusion, although the myocardium at risk is the same, the extent of the infarction is less.

Sudden death

A large proportion of patients with coronary artery disease die suddenly (Table 3.19) without evidence of acute myocardial infarction *(216)*. The presumption is that death is due to an arrhythmia, usually ventricular tachycardia deteriorating into fibrillation. The arrhythmia may arise in the presence of either an acute event in the coronary arteries (an unstable plaque) or in severe atheromatous coronary artery disease. Many factors contribute to arrhythmias, including stimulation of the autonomic nervous system and alterations in the concentration of many substances in the blood and within the cell, for example, magnesium concentration and the intracellular accumulation of lipids.

Table 3.19　Causes of sudden death (age 19 – 69 years)

	All (%) (n = 322)	Men (%) (n = 238)	Women (%) (n = 84)
Ischaemic heart disease	60	65	41
Respiratory disease	18	14	27
Non-ischaemic cardiac disease	8	6	12
Central nervous system disease	4	3	8
Aortic aneurysm	3	4	1
Gastrointestinal haemorrhage	2	4	2
Cause unknown	3	3	6
Alcohol-related	3	1	2

Thomas et al., Br Med J 1988; **297**: 1453

A major factor may be the extracellular accumulation of potassium in the ischaemic myocardium. The margin of a myocardial infarct is now known to be sharp so that normal myocardial cells being perfused at a potassium concentration of 4.5 mmol.l^{-1} lie adjacent to cells with an extracellular potassium concentration of up to 10 mmol.l^{-1}. Thus, there is a gradient between the high extracellular potassium concentration in the middle of the infarcted area and normal tissue. Such an electrical inhomogeneity within the heart may provide the electrical basis of arrhythmias; the 'trigger' may be stimulation of the sympathetic nervous system or sudden alterations in the extracellular potassium concentration for normal tissue. Recent work shows that the plasma potassium concentration alters from minute to minute, particularly with exercise.

Sudden death should not be equated or confused with acute myocardial infarction (216) as their circumstances and underlying mechanisms may be very different. Reports vary greatly on the incidence of coronary thrombosis in patients with sudden death (24,74,75), which almost certainly reflects the different definitions of sudden death, exclusion of selected groups of patients and different techniques for pathological examination of the post-mortem specimen. If sudden death is defined as the death of a person who was well during the previous 24 hours in one study, the proportion of patients with recognized myocardial infarction will differ. Six hours is long in terms of the development of an infarction, yet post-mortem techniques cannot easily detect myocardial infarction if it was present for less than approximately three hours. Studies of patients who have survived cardiac resuscitation indicate that only a small proportion (17%) develop a myocardial infarct.

A common feature in most patients who die suddenly is severe coronary artery disease. It is likely, therefore, that many of these deaths are due to an arrhythmia which may have been induced by the ionic events (described above) which accompany a short period of myocardial ischaemia. One report indicates a high incidence of unstable atheromatous plaques and thrombosis in patients with coronary artery disease, but it may be that, in this study, there was a greater proportion of patients with early myocardial infarction compared to other studies.

The clinical implication is that agents known to prevent or interfere with the alleged mechanisms of myocardial infarction may not necessarily be effective in the prevention of sudden death. Agents which terminate arrhythmias or interfere with the early mechanisms of ischaemia similarly may not be effective in preventing myocardial infarction.

There is, thus far, little knowledge of the anatomy and pathology of atheroma in the coronary arteries which may be associated with sudden death. A simple possibility is that, where a coronary artery is totally occluded and no collaterals are present, sudden death is more common. Thus, in a patient with angina, the first ischaemic episode may be less damaging because there has been time for the development of collaterals which limit the severity and extent of the ischaemic episode. A congenital presence of collaterals may also be protective.

Syndrome X

The term 'syndrome X' was first used by Kemp *(221)* in an editorial discussing a report on angina pectoris in which a specific group of patients in a table was called 'X', and the label was later popularized by Opherk and colleagues *(222)*. Syndrome X describes an entity with three features:

Patients experience chest pain which is not readily distinguishable from angina pectoris.

Investigation by coronary angiography shows no abnormality of the large coronary arteries; it is important to appreciate that coronary angiograms only visualize coronary arteries of greater than 400 μm in diameter, and histological examination of biopsies provides information on vessels less than 150 μm in diameter.

The exercise test shows features (ST-segment depression) which, in patients with atheromatous obstructive coronary artery disease, are considered characteristic of myocardial ischaemia.

The third criterion is not always present in patients with normal coronary arteries and chest pain. Positive exercise tests have been reported in 0 to 69% of patients *(223)*.

Syndrome X is here defined as the presence of chest pain suggestive of angina pectoris, normal coronary arteries on angiography and a positive exercise test (presence of ST-segment depression) in the absence of any other known disease of the heart. Numerous workers have studied the syndrome, but many have included patients who do not fulfil all criteria, in particular, a positive exercise test. Abnormalities in ventricular function, perfusion, lactate production and histology have been reported *(223)*. Some studies were clearly describing a cardiomyopathy rather than syndrome X, and other studies have assumed that ST-segment depression is synonymous with myocardial ischaemia.

This present author's work has been directed at understanding the origin of the chest pain and measuring coronary sinus oxygen concentrations during an atrial-pacing test. An interesting observation is that, in a large proportion of these patients, chest pain can be induced by manipulation of a catheter in the right atrium *(224)*. In a study involving 11 patients *(61)*, all but two did not develop a sustained fall of coronary sinus oxygen saturation during atrial pacing, despite the appearance of ST-segment depression on ECG, and the onset of chest pain was similar to exercise-induced chest pain. In two patients, the fall in coronary sinus oxygen saturation was similar to that in patients with obstructive coronary artery disease. These two patients presumably had small-vessel disease which was not detectable by coronary angiography, an obstruction in vessels of a diameter less than 400μm. There is as yet no direct evidence of such an abnormality.

> The multitude of different findings in syndrome X suggests that the entity is not a single disease, but an inhomogeneous group of diseases.

Several mechanisms have been put forward, and speculative abnormalities include small-vessel disease (with reduction of cardiac reserve), a 'steal' phenomenon, myocardial cell abnormalities, epi-endocardial redistribution of blood flow and altered responses to acetylcholine or EDRF.

The most widely held view is that syndrome X is a disorder of myocardial microvasculature. This appears to be true in a minority of patients who often have conduction defects within the heart and may be in early cardiomyopathy. Follow-up of these patients has shown that cardiomyopathy develops in patients who have both syndrome X and conduction disturbances, and abnormalities of the microvasculature are present in some forms of cardiomyopathy. The prognosis for this subgroup may be less positive.

Some workers have suggested that patients with normal coronary arteries and anginal symptoms often have a limited coronary flow reserve *(225)*, but almost none of these patients had ST-segment depression on exercise or during the episode of chest pain. Data were obtained from patients under cardiac catheterization to distinguish those who developed pain during an atrial-pacing test in the presence of ergonovine. However, there were no responses from the normal control group to this procedure. Pain during an atrial-pacing test is problematical to evaluate because of the difficulty in distinguishing the chest sensations associated with pacing from the development of anginal pain.

The pathophysiology of syndrome X is not understood. A proportion of these patients may have a true ischaemia which more appropriately should be termed 'microvascular angina'. The majority appear not to have myocardial ischaemia; other reasons must be considered for the presence of the ST-segment changes often mistaken as evidence of ischaemia. One possibility is that these patients have a minor difference in myocardial structure, perhaps in the anatomical relationship between capillaries and myocytes or in the channels in cells so that, with an increase in heart rate or when other signs of stress are present, potassium accumulates in the clefts between cells. This may cause the changes seen on ECG and precipitate chest pain. Another possibility is that the normal function of channels involved in ionic exchange is altered by hormonal factors.

An important consequence of such an hypothesis is that the ST-segment changes seen on ambulatory ECG monitoring should not be assumed to be the consequence of obstructive coronary artery disease, and 24-hour ST-segment depression is not a measure of the 'total ischaemic burden' unless other evidence of ischaemia is obtained. Positive exercise tests in a small proportion of the population are to be expected (for reasons not yet known) and should not carry a poor prognosis.

Silent ischaemia

Silent ischaemia is a topical and fashionable concept, although the idea is not new. Physicians many years ago identified patients with evidence of ischaemia on ECG and no chest pain. Silent myocardial infarction is said to occur in approximately 25% of cases *(209)*, in the opinion of this present author, a suspect figure because patients often cannot recall chest pain, and infarction without chest pain is almost unknown. Silent ischaemia was popularized by the availability of 24-hour ECG monitoring *(210,211)*. The initial observation was the occurrence of many episodes of ST-segment depression without chest pain because either, at that instant, other factors suppressed the pain (altered pain threshold) or pain-receptor stimuli were absent.

The concept of silent ischaemia was then extended to include the idea that multiple episodes of ischaemia could lead to a sustained abnormality of myocardial contraction (stuttering ischaemia and stunned myocardium), necrosis of cells as a result of repetitive ischaemia and an increased risk of death. The concept of 'total ischaemic burden' emerged *(228)*.

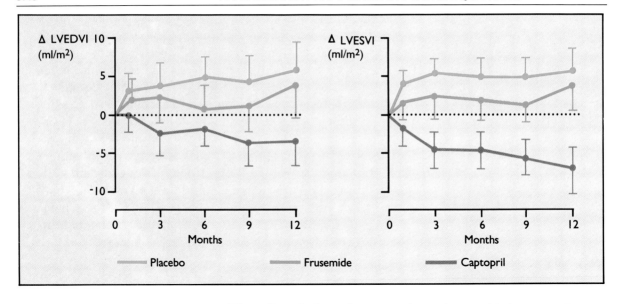

Figure 3.10 An increase in ventricular volume after acute myocardial infarction can be prevented by the early use of an ACE inhibitor (captopril). From Sharpe *et al.*, *Lancet* 1988; i: 255-9.

That silent ischaemia occurs in patients with known atheromatous disease of the coronary arteries is well documented. Mild coronary artery disease is a predictor of death from coronary artery disease. The key questions are whether the total ischaemic burden contributes to myocardial damage and whether silent ischaemia is an independent marker of coronary risk. Recent studies suggest that, as expected, patients with silent ischaemia have a prognosis in-between those with silent and overt ischaemia, and normal subjects *(227)*.

The problem is confounded by the difficulty of diagnosing ischaemia. Early work wherein patients underwent coronary angiography showed that approximately half of the patients had atheroma and the prognosis was worse if a positive exercise test was found *(226, 229)*. This may have been due to a poor prognosis for those with atheroma, but a good prognosis for those with changes on ECG but without atheroma. Thus, a mixed population may account for the in-between prognosis for silent ischaemia *(227)*. One study *(230)* showed that silent ischaemia occurs in those with overt ischaemia but adds little to the diagnosis. Silent ischaemia on its own is rare.

ST-segment depression or elevation on ECG during exercise is often interpreted as an indication of myocardial ischaemia. This is usually true in patients with angina pectoris and atheromatous disease of the coronary arteries as coronary blood flow has been shown to be reduced at the time of the appearance of angina. However, this interpretation should not be applied to ST-segment changes in other circumstances. Numerous medical conditions are known to cause so-called false-positive changes. These include hypertension, hypertrophy, the use of digoxin and circumstances in which catecholamines are raised. Depression of the ST segment can be detected on 24-hour Holter monitoring in normal subjects during exercise and under stressful conditions.

The ECG is the sum of electrical events in the whole heart as measured where the applied electrodes are positioned. ST-segment depression is attributed partly to a reduction in the amplitude of the action-potential plateau period and partly to currents during diastole. What is essential is that there are potential differences between different parts of the myocardium.

Most of the changes on myocardial action potential during ischaemia can be accounted for by the accumulation of potassium in the extracellular space and the development of acidosis. The conditions under which false-positive ST-segment depression arises are characterized by either alteration of the function of the sodium pump, changes of contractility, increases of heart rate or abnormal anatomy of the myocardium, circumstances wherein potassium is likely to accumulate in the spaces between cells randomly throughout the myocardium. Increases of heart rate are known to cause a transient loss of potassium from myocardial tissue, and the same phenomenon has been demonstrated in man in the absence of any obstruction of the coronary arteries.

Thus, there is a substantial danger that use of the changes on ECG will detect a large proportion of patients who do not have atheromatous coronary artery disease and who have a good prognosis. These patients may then be subjected to the discomfort, cost and risk of coronary angiography. This also applies to use of the exercise test and even to use of 24-hour Holter monitoring. Silent ischaemia, although a popular concept *(228)*, may be dangerously misleading if not carefully considered in the light of other evidence for the presence of atheromatous obstructive coronary artery disease.

Conclusion

The entity 'ischaemic heart disease' encompasses a large number of clinical syndromes which account for considerable morbidity and mortality. The underlying pathology is the presence of atheroma in the wall of the coronary arteries. The enlargement results in the formation of plaques. The growth of these plaques involves the interaction between endothelial cells, smooth muscle cells, monocytes, platelets and macrophages, and the constituents of the blood, notably lipid and cholesterol. The clinical syndromes associated with ischaemic heart disease are rarely related to the static effects of a plaque but to the dynamic changes brought about either by rupture of the plaque or the attachment and aggregation of platelets to the plaque.

The last decade has seen major advances not only in understanding the pathology of ischaemic heart disease but also in its treatment. Thrombolytic therapy for the treatment of acute myocardial infarction is now standard practice. Angioplasty and coronary artery surgery have been available for some time.

There are several major directions for future research. In the coronary arteries, it is important to understand the interaction between cell types and those factors which bring about proliferation of smooth muscle. In the heart itself, there is a need for knowledge of how hypertrophy of the myocyte is controlled and how the shape and architecture of the heart are changed after infarction or in response to an increase of preload and afterload. When the heart enlarges, there is considerable slippage of myocytes. The mechanism is as yet unknown.

It is a truism that prevention is better than cure. For the foreseeable future, so many people will be afflicted by the consequences of ischaemic heart disease that it is essential to continue research into and seek treatment for the numerous manifestations of atheromatous coronary artery disease. Prevention is possible, but the results of recent trials have been less impressive than anticipated. New approaches are needed for the identification of those who develop atheroma in the coronary arteries and for the early detection of coronary disease. This would allow the identification of those at risk and the direction of resources and treatment to that particular group. At the same time, it is reasonable to give advice to the general population to stop smoking, follow a varied diet, avoid obesity, treat hypertension (in order to prevent strokes) and participate in some form of exercise.

References

1. Hearse DJ, Yellon DM, Downey JM. Can beta-blockers limit myocardial infarct size? *Eur Heart J* 1986; 11: 925-30.

2. Fitzgerald JD. By what means might beta-blockers prolong life after acute myocardial infarction? *Eur Heart J* 1987; 8: 945-51.

3. Beta-blocker Heart Attack Trial Research Group. A randomized trial of propranolol in patients with acute myocardial infarction. *JAMA* 1982; 247: 1707-14.

4. Norwegian Multicenter Study Group. Timolol-induced reduction in mortality and reinfarction in patients with acute myocardial infarction. *N Engl J Med* 1981; 304: 801-7.

5. ISIS-1 (First International Study of Infarct Survival) Collaborative Group. Ischaemic heart disease. Randomised trial of intravenous atenolol among 16,027 cases of suspected acute myocardial infarction: ISIS-1. *Lancet* 1986; ii: 57-65.

6. Yusuf S, Peto R, Lewis J, Collins R, Sleight P. Beta-blockade during and after myocardial infarction: An overview of the randomised trials. *Prog Cardiovasc Dis* 1985; 27: 335-71.

7. Yusuf S, Collins R, Peto R, et al. Intravenous and intracoronary fibrinolytic therapy in acute myocardial infarction: Overview of results on mortality, reinfarction and side-effects from 33 randomised controlled trials. *Eur Heart J* 1985; 6: 556-83.

8. GISSI Study. Effectiveness of intravenous thrombolytic treatment in acute myocardial infarction. *Lancet* 1986; i: 397-401.

9. ISIS-2 Collaborative Group. Randomised trial of intravenous streptokinase, oral aspirin, both, or neither among 17,187 cases of suspected acute myocardial infarction: ISIS-2. *Lancet* 1988; ii: 349-60.

10. AIMS Trial Study Group. Effect of intravenous APSAC on mortality after acute myocardial infarction: Preliminary report of a placebo-controlled trial. *Lancet* 1988; i: 545-9.

11. Wilcox RG, Olsson CG, Skene AM, Von der Lippe G, Jensen G, Hampton JR. Trial of tissue plasminogen activator for mortality reduction in acute myocardial infarction. *Lancet* 1988; ii: 526-30.

12. The ISAM Study Group. A prospective trial of intravenous streptokinase in acute myocardial infarction (ISAM). Mortality, morbidity, and infarct size at 21 days. *N Engl J Med* 1986; 314: 1465-71.

13. Hearse DJ, Yellon DM. The 'border zone' in evolving myocardial infarction: Controversy or confusion? *Am J Cardiol* 1981; 49 (6): 1321-34.

14. Hearse DJ, Yellon DM, eds. *Therapeutic Approaches to Myocardial Infarct Size Limitation.* New York: Raven Press, 1984.

15. Gruntzig AR, Senning A, Siegenthaler WE. Non-operative dilatation of coronary-artery stenosis: Percutaneous transluminal coronary angioplasty. *N Engl J Med* 1979; 301: 61-8.

16. Ganz W, Buchbinder N, Marcus H, et al. Intracoronary thrombolysis in evolving myocardial infarction. *Am Heart J* 1981; 101: 4-13.

17. Mathey DG, Kuck KH, Tilsner V, Krebber HJ, Bleifeld W. Non-surgical coronary artery recanalisation after acute transluminal infarction. *Circulation* 1981; 67: 489-97.

18. Rentrop KP, Blanke H, Karsch KR, Kaiser H, Kostering H, Leitz K. Selective intracoronary thrombolysis in acute myocardial infarction and unstable angina pectoris. *Circulation* 1981; 63: 307-17.

19. Eaton LW, Weiss JL, Bulkley BH, Garrison JB, Weisfeldt ML. Regional cardiac dilatation after acute myocardial infarction. *N Engl J Med* 1979; 300: 57-62.

20. Armstrong A, Duncan B, Oliver MF. Natural history of acute coronary heart attacks. A community study. *Br Heart J* 1972; 34: 67-80.

21. Tunstall-Pedoe H. Heart disease mortality. *Br Med J* 1989; 298: 751.

22. Simons LA. Interrelations of lipids and lipoproteins with coronary artery disease mortality in 19 countries. *Am J Cardiol* 1986; 57: 5G-10G.

23. Stehbens WE. An appraisal of the epidemic rise of coronary heart disease and its decline. *Lancet* 1987; i: 606-10.

24. Thomas AC, Knapman PA, Krikler DM, Davies MJ. Community study of the causes of 'natural' sudden death. *Br Med J* 1988; 297: 1453-6.

25. Kannel WB, Neaton JD, Wentworth D. Overall and coronary heart disease mortality rates in relation to major risk factors in 325,348 men screened for the MRFIT. *Am Heart J* 1986; 112: 825-36.

26. The Pooling Project Research Group. Relationship of blood pressure, serum cholesterol, smoking habit, relative weight and ECG abnormalities to incidence of major coronary events. Final report of the Pooling Project. *J Chronic Dis* 1978; 31: 201-306.

27. Anderson KM, Castelli WP, Levy D. Cholesterol and mortality. 30 years of follow-up from the Framingham Study. *JAMA* 1987; 257: 2176-80.

28. Fleck A. Latitude and ischaemic heart disease. *Lancet* 1989; ii: 613.

29. Shaper AG, Pocock SJ, Phillips AN, Walker M. Identifying men at high risk of heart attacks: Strategy for use in general practice. *Br Med J* 1986; 293: 474-9.

30. Taylor WC, Pass TM, Shepard DS, Komaroff AL. Cholesterol reduction and life expectancy. *Ann Intern Med* 1987; 106: 605-14.

31. McCormick J, Skrabanek P. Coronary heart disease is not preventable by population interventions. *Lancet* 1988; ii: 839-41.

32. Veterans Administration Cooperative Study Group on Antihypertensive Agents. Effects of treatment on morbidity in hypertension. II. Results in patients with diastolic blood pressure averaging 90 through 114 mm Hg. *JAMA* 1970; 213: 1143-52.

33. Berglund G, Sannerstedt R, Andersson O, et al. Coronary heart disease after treatment of hypertension. *Lancet* 1978; i: 1-6.

34. Hypertension Detection and Follow-up Program Cooperative Group. The effect of treatment on mortality in 'mild' hypertension. Results of the Hypertension Detection and Follow-up Program. *N Engl J Med* 1982; 307: 976-9.

35. Helgeland A. Treatment of mild hypertension: A five-year controlled drug trial. The Oslo Study. *Am J Med* 1980; 69: 725-32.

36. The Australian Therapeutic Trial in Mild Hypertension. Report by the Management Committee. *Lancet* 1980; i: 1261-9.

37. Medical Research Council Working Party, Northwick Park Hospital, Harrow, UK. MRC Trial of treatment of mild hypertension: Principal results. *Br Med J* 1985; 291: 97-105.

38. Coller BS. Platelets and thrombolytic therapy. *N Engl J Med* 1990; 322: 33-42.

39. Amery A, Birkenhager W, Brixko R, et al. Efficacy of antihypertensive treatment according to age, sex, blood pressure, and previous cardiovascular disease in patients over the age of 60. *Lancet* 1986; ii: 590-2.

40. IPPPSH Collaborative Group. Cardiovascular risk and risk factors in a randomised trial of treatment based on the beta-blocker oxprenolol. *Br Med J* 1989; 298: 379-92.

41. Coope J, Warrender TS. Randomised trial of hypertension in elderly patients in primary care. *Br Med J* 1986; 293: 1145-51.

42. Wilhelmsen L, Berglund G, Elmfeldt D, et al. on behalf of the Heart Attack Primary Prevention in Hypertension Research Group. Beta-blockers versus diuretics in hypertensive men: Main results from the HAPPHY trial. *J Hypertens* 1987; 5: 561-72.

43. Brett AS. Treating hypercholesterolaemia: How should practicing physicians interpret the published data from patients? *N Engl J Med* 1989; 321: 676-80.

44. Oliver MF. Prevention of coronary heart disease – propaganda, promises, problems, and prospects. *Circulation* 1986; 73: 1-9.

45. Leaf A. Management of hypercholesterolemia: Are preventive interventions advisable? *N Engl J Med* 1989; 321: 680-4.

46. Corday E, Ryden L. Why some physicians have concerns about the cholesterol awareness program. *J Am Coll Cardiol* 1989; 13: 497-502.

47. Mann GV. Diet-heart: End of an era. *N Engl J Med* 1977; 297: 644-50.

48. Ahrens EH. Dietary fats and coronary heart disease: Unfinished business. *Lancet* 1979; ii: 1345-8.

49. Gunning-Schepers LJ, Barendregt JJ, Van der Maas PJ. Population interventions reassessed. *Lancet* 1989; i:479-81.

50. Fries JF, Green LW, Levine S. Health promotion and the compression of morbidity. *Lancet* 1989; i:481-3.

51. Smith WCS, Kenicer MB, Maryon-Davis A, Evans AE, Yarnell J. Blood cholesterol: Is population screening warranted in the UK? *Lancet* 1989; i: 372-3.

52. The British Cardiac Society Working Party on Coronary Prevention: Conclusions and recommendations. *Br Heart J* 1987; 57: 188-9.

53. Martin MJ, Hulley SB, Browner WS, Kuller LH, Wentworth D. Serum cholesterol, blood pressure, and mortality: Implications from a cohort of 361,662 men. *Lancet* 1986; ii: 933-6.

54. Isles CG, Hole DJ, Hawthorne VM, Lever AF. Plasma cholesterol, coronary heart disease and cancer in the Renfrew and Paisley survey. *Br Med J* 1989; 298: 920-4.

55. Lipid Research Clinics Program. The Lipid Research Clinics Coronary Primary Prevention Trial results. 1. Reduction in incidence of coronary heart disease, and 2. The relationship of reduction in incidence of coronary heart disease to cholesterol-lowering. *JAMA* 1984; 251: 351-74.

56. Frick MH, Elo O, Haapa K, et al. Helsinki heart study: Primary-prevention trial with gemfibrozil in middle-aged men with dyslipidemia. Safety of treatment, changes in risk factors, and incidence of coronary heart disease. N Engl J Med 1987; 317: 1237-45.

57. Committee of principal investigators. A cooperative trial in the primary prevention of ischaemic heart disease using clofibrate. Br Heart J 1978; 40: 1069-118.

58. Blankenhorn DH, Nessim SA, Johnson RL, SanMarco ME, Azen SP, Cashen-Hemphill L. Beneficial effects of combined colestipol-niacin therapy on coronary atherosclerosis and coronary venous bypass grafts. JAMA 1987; 257: 3233-40.

59. Lichtlen PR, Hugenholtz P, Rafflenbeul W, Hecker H, Jost S, Deckers JW, on behalf of the INTACT group of investigators. Retardation of angiographic progression of coronary artery disease by nifedipine. Lancet 1990; 335: 1109-1113.

60. World Health Organization European Collaborative Group. European Collaborative Trial of Multifactorial Prevention of Coronary Heart Disease: Final report on the 6-year results. Lancet 1986; i: 869-72.

61. Crake T, Crean P, Shapiro LM, Canepa-Anson R, Poole-Wilson PA. Continuous recording of coronary sinus oxygen saturation during atrial pacing in patients with and without coronary artery disease or with syndrome X. Br Heart J 1987; 57: 67.

62. Marcus ML. The Coronary Circulation in Health and Disease. New York: McGraw-Hill, 1983.

63. Schaper W. The Pathophysiology of Myocardial Perfusion. Amsterdam and New York: Elsevier/North Holland Biomedical Press, 1979.

64. Vanhoutte PM, Shimokawa H. Endothelium-derived relaxing factor and coronary spasm. Circulation 1989; 80: 1-9.

65. Neely JR, Morgan HE. Relation between carbohydrate and lipid metabolism and the energy balance of the heart. Ann Rev Physiol 1974; 36: 413-59.

66. Neely JR, Rovetto MJ, Whitmer JT, Morgan HE. Effects of ischemia on function and metabolism of the isolated working rat heart. Am J Physiol 1973; 225: 651.

67. Neely JR, Whitmer JT, Rovetto MJ. Effect of coronary blood flow on glycolytic flux and intracellular pH in isolated rat hearts. Circ Res 1975; 37: 733-41.

68. Crake T, Crean P, Shapiro L, Rickards AF, Poole-Wilson PA. Coronary sinus pH during percutaneous transluminal angioplasty: Early development of acidosis during myocardial ischaemia in man. Br Heart J 1987; 58: 110-5.

69. Chierchia S, Brunelli C, Simonetti I, Lazzari M, Maseri A. Sequence of events in angina at rest: Primary reduction in coronary flow. Circulation 1980; 61: 759-68.

70. Braunwald E, Kloner RA. The stunned myocardium: Prolonged, postischemic ventricular dysfunction. Circulation 1982; 66: 1146-9.

71. Poole-Wilson PA. What causes cell death? In: Hearse DJ, Yellon DM, eds. Therapeutic Approaches to Myocardial Infarct Size Limitation. New York: Raven Press, 1984; 43-60.

72. Kloner RA, Fishbein MC, Lew H, Maroko PR, Braunwald E. Mummification of the infarcted myocardium by high-dose corticosteroids. Circulation 1978; 57: 56-63.

73. Cohn PF. Silent myocardial ischaemia: Dimensions of the problem in patients with and without angina. Am J Med 1986; 80 (Suppl 4c): 3-8.

74. Davies MJ, Thomas A. Thrombosis and acute coronary artery lesions in sudden cardiac death. N Engl J Med 1984; 310: 1137-40.

75. Davies MJ, Thomas AC. Plaque fissuring – the cause of acute myocardial infarction, sudden ischaemic death, and crescendo angina (review of 60 refs). Br Heart J 1985; 53: 363-73.

76. McCord JM, Roy RS. The pathophysiology of superoxide: Roles in inflammation and ischaemia. Can J Physiol Pharmacol 1982; 60: 1346-52.

77. Allen DG, Morris PG, Orchard CH, Pirolo JS. A nuclear magnetic resonance study of metabolism in the ferret heart during hypoxia and inhibition of glycolysis. J Physiol 1985; 361: 185-204.

78. Jacobus WE, Pores IH, Lucas SK, Clayton HK, Weisfeldt ML, Flaherty JT. The role of intracellular pH in the control of normal and ischaemic myocardial contractility. In: Nuccitelli R, Deamer DW, eds. Intracellular pH. New York: Alan Liss, 1983: 537-65.

79. Ellis D, Noireaud J. Intracellular pH in sheep Purkinje fibres and ferret papillary muscles during hypoxia and recovery. J Physiol 1987; 383: 125-41.

80. Cobbe SM, Poole-Wilson PA. Tissue acidosis in myocardial hypoxia. J Mol Cell Cardiol 1980; 12: 761-70.

81. Cobbe SM, Poole-Wilson PA. Continuous coronary sinus and arterial pH monitoring during pacing-induced ischaemia in coronary artery disease. Br Heart J 1982; 47: 369-74.

82. Serruys PW, Wijns W, Van den Brond M, et al. Left ventricular performance, regional blood flow, wall motion and lactate metabolism during transluminal angioplasty. Circulation 1984; 70: 25-36.

83. Harding DP, Poole-Wilson PA. Calcium exchange in rabbit myocardium during and after hypoxia: Effect of temperature and substrate. Cardiovasc Res 1980; 14(8): 435-45.

84. Sayen JJ, Sheldon WF, Pierce G, Kuo PT. Polarographic oxygen, the epicardial electrocardiogram and muscle contraction in experimental acute regional ischaemia of the left ventricle. Circ Res 1958; 6: 779-98.

85. Braasch W, Gudbjarnson S, Puri PS, Ravens KG, Bing RJ. Early changes in energy metabolism in the myocardium following acute coronary artery occlusion in anaesthetized dogs. Circ Res 1968; 23: 429-38.

86. Gudbjarnson S, Mathes P, Ravens KG. Functional compartmentalisation of ATP and creatine phosphate in heart muscle. J Mol Cell Cardiol 1970; 1: 325-39.

87. Wollenberger A, Krause EG. Metabolic control characteristics of the acutely ischemic myocardium. Am J Cardiol 1968; 22: 349-59.

88. Tennant R, Wiggers CJ. The effect of coronary occlusion on myocardial contraction. Am J Physiol 1935; 112: 351-61.

89. Tennant R. Factors concerned in the arrest of contraction in an ischaemic myocardial area. Am J Physiol 1935; 113: 677-82.

90. Donaldson RM, Taggart P, Bennett JG, Rickards AF. Study of electrophysiological ischemic events during coronary angioplasty. Texas Heart Inst J 1984; 11: 23-30.

91. Poole-Wilson PA, Fleetwood G, Cobbe SM. Early contractile failure in myocardial ischaemia – role of acidosis. In: Refsum H, Jynge P, Mjos OD, eds. Myocardial Ischaemia and Protection. Edinburgh: Churchill Livingstone, 1983; 9-17.

92. Apstein CS, Mueller M, Hood WB. Ventricular contracture and compliance changes with global ischaemia and reperfusion, and their effect on coronary resistance changes in the rat. Circ Res 1977; 41: 206-17.

93. Arnold G, Kosche F, Miessner E, Neitzert A, Lochner W. The importance of the perfusion pressure in the coronary arteries for the contractility and the oxygen consumption of the heart. Pflügers Archiv 1968; 299: 339-56.

94. Cobbe SM, Parker DJ, Poole-Wilson PA. Tissue and coronary venous pH in ischemic canine myocardium. Clin Cardiol 1982; 5: 153-6.

95. Allen DG, Orchard CH. The effect of pH on intracellular calcium transients in mammalian cardiac muscle. J Physiol 1983; 335: 555-67.

96. Kubler W, Katz AM. Mechanism of early 'pump' failure of the ischemic heart: Possible role of adenosine triphosphate depletion and inorganic phosphate accumulation. Am J Cardiol 1977; 40: 467-71.

97. Kirkels JH, van Echteld CJA, Ruigrok TJC. Intracellular magnesium during myocardial ischemia and reperfusion: Possible consequences for postischemic recovery. J Mol Cell Cardiol 1989; 21: 1209-18.

98. Kentish JC. The effect of inorganic phosphate and creatine phosphate on force production in skinned muscle from rat ventricle. J Physiol 1985; 370: 585-604.

99. Bricknell OL, Opie LH. Effects of substrates on tissue metabolic changes in the isolated rat heart during underperfusion and on release of lactate dehydrogenase. *Circ Res* 1978; 43: 102-15.

100. Higgins TJC, Allsopp D, Bailey PJ, D'Souza EDA. The relationship between glycolysis, fatty acid metabolism and membrane integrity in neonatal myocytes. *J Mol Cell Cardiol* 1981; 13: 599-615.

101. Kentish JC, Allen DG. Is force production in the myocardium dependent on the free energy change? *Am J Physiol* 1979; 236(1): R21-39.

102. Kammermeier H, Schmidt P, Jungling E. Free energy change of ATP hydrolysis: A causal factor of early hypoxic failure of the myocardium? *J Mol Cell Cardiol* 1982; 14: 267-77.

103. Weiss J, Shine KI. Extracellular K+ accumulation during early myocardial ischemia. Implications for arrhythmogenesis. *J Mol Cell Cardiol* 1981; 13: 699-704.

104. Hirche HJ, Franz C, Bos L, Bissig R, Lang R, Schramm M. Myocardial extracellular K+ and H+ increase and noradrenaline release as possible cause of early arrhythmias following acute coronary artery occlusion in pigs. *J Mol Cell Cardiol* 1980; 12: 579-94.

105. Hill JL, Gettes LS. Effect of acute coronary artery occlusion on local myocardial extracellular K+ activity in swine. *Circulation* 1980; 61: 68-78.

106. Wiegand V, Guggi M, Meesmann W, Kessler M, Greitschus F. Extracellular potassium activity changes in the canine myocardium. *Cardiovasc Res* 1979; 13: 297-302.

107. Weiss J, Shine KI. (K+)o accumulation and electrophysiological alterations during early myocardial ischaemia. *Am J Physiol* 1982; 243: H318-27.

108. Webb SC, Fleetwood GG, Montgomery RAP, Poole-Wilson PA. Absence of a relationship between extracellular potassium accumulation and contractile failure in the ischemic or hypoxic rabbit heart. In: Dhalla NS, Hearse DJ, eds. *Advances in Myocardiology, Volume 6.* New York, London: Plenum Medical Book Co; 1984: 405-15.

109. Webb SC, Rickards AF, Poole-Wilson PA. Coronary sinus potassium concentration recorded during coronary angioplasty. *Br Heart J* 1983; 50: 146-8.

110. Gaspardone A, Shine KI, Seabrooke SR, Poole-Wilson PA. Potassium loss from rabbit myocardium during hypoxia; evidence for passive efflux linked to anion extrusion. *J Mol Cell Cardiol* 1986; 18: 389-99.

111. Kleber AG. Extracellular potassium accumulation in acute myocardial ischemia. *J Mol Cell Cardiol* 1984; 16(5): 389-94.

112. Kleber AG. Resting membrane potential, extracellular potassium activity and intracellular sodium activity during acute global ischaemia in isolated perfused guinea pig hearts. *Circ Res* 1983; 52: 442-50.

113. Noma A. ATP-regulated K+ channels in cardiac muscle. *Nature* 1983; 305: 147-8.

114. Jennings RB, Hawkins HK, Lowe JE, Hill MC, Klotman S, Reimer KA. Relation between high-energy phosphate and lethal injury in myocardial ischemia in the dog. *Am J Pathol* 1978; 92: 187-214.

115. Jennings RB, Ganote CE, Reimer KA. Ischaemic tissue injury. *Am J Pathol* 1975; 81: 179-98.

116. Kloner RA, Przyklenk K, Whittaker P. Deleterious effects of oxygen radicals in ischemia/reperfusion: Resolved and unresolved issues. *Circulation* 1989; 80: 1115-27.

117. Post JA, Lamers JMJ, Ten Cate FJ, Van der Giessen WJ, Verkleij AJ. Sarcolemmal destabilization and destruction after ischaemic and reperfusion and its relation with long-term recovery of regional ventricular function in pigs. *Eur Heart J* 1987; 8: 423-30.

118. Post JA, Leunissen-Bijvelt J, Riugrok TJC, Verkleij AJ. Ultrastructural changes of sarcolemma and mitochondria in the isolated rabbit heart during ischaemia and reperfusion. *Biochem Biophys Acta* 1985; 845: 119-23.

119. Steenbergen C, Murphy E, Levy L, London RE. Elevation in cytosolic free calcium concentration early in myocardial ischemia in perfused rat heart. *Circ Res* 1987; 60: 700-7.

120. Marban E, Kitakaze M, Kusuoka H, Porterfield JK, Yue DT. Intracellular free-calcium concentration measured with 19F NMR spectroscopy in intact ferret hearts. *Proc Natl Acad Sci* 1987; 84: 6005-9.

121. Lee H-C, Mohabir R, Smith N, Franz MR, Clusin WT. Effect of ischemia on calcium-dependent fluorescence transients in rabbit hearts containing indo 1. Correlation with monophasic action potentials and contraction. *Circulation* 1988; 78: 1047-59.

122. Lee H-C, Smith N, Mohabir R, Clusin WT. Cytosolic calcium transients from the beating mammalian heart. *Proc Natl Acad Sci* 1987; 84: 7793-7.

123. Allen DG, Lee JA, Smith GL. The consequences of simulated ischaemia on intracellular Ca2+ and tension in isolated ferret ventricular muscle. *J Physiol* 1989; 410: 297-323.

124. Steenbergen C, Jennings RB. Relationship between lysophospholipid accumulation and plasma membrane injury during total in vitro ischaemia in dog heart. *J Mol Cell Cardiol* 1984; 16: 605-21.

125. Reimer KA, Jennings RB, Cobb FR, *et al*. Animal models for protecting ischaemic myocardium: Results of the NHLBI cooperative study. Comparison of unconscious and conscious dog models. *Circ Res* 1985; 56: 651-65.

126. Schaper W. Experimental infarcts and the microcirculation. In: Hearse DJ, Yellon DM, eds. *Therapeutic Approaches to Myocardial Infarct Size Limitation.* New York: Raven Press, 1984: 79-90.

127. Hearse DJ. Reperfusion of the ischemic myocardium. *J Mol Cell Cardiol* 1977; 9: 605-16.

128. Yamazaki S, Fujibayashi Y, Rajogopalan RE, Meerbaum S, Corday E. Effects of staged versus sudden reperfusion after acute coronary occlusion in the dog. *J Am Coll Cardiol* 1986; 7: 564-72.

129. Davies GJ, Cherchia S, Maseri A. Prevention of myocardial infarction by very early treatment with intracoronary streptokinase. *N Engl J Med* 1984; 311: 1488-92.

130. Hackett D, Davies G, Cherchia S, Maseri A. Intermittent coronary occlusion in acute myocardial infarction: Value of combined thrombolytic and vasodilator therapy. *N Engl J Med* 1987; 317: 1055-9.

131. Kloner RA, Ganote CE, Whalen DA, Jennings RB. Effects of a transient period of ischemia on myocardial cells. II. Fine structure during the first few minutes of reflow. *Am J Pathol* 1974; 74: 399-422.

132. Fleetwood G, Poole-Wilson PA. Diastolic coronary resistance in the isolated rabbit heart during and after ischaemia: Contribution of extracellular forces. *Cardiovasc Res* 1986; 20: 883-90.

133. Humphrey SM, Gavin JB, Herdson PB. The relationship of ischemic contracture to vascular reperfusion in the isolated rat heart. *J Mol Cell Cardiol* 1980; 12: 1397-1406.

134. Powers ER, DiBona DR, Powell Jr WJ. Myocardial cell volume and coronary resistance during diminished coronary perfusion. *Am J Physiol* 1984; 247: H467-77.

135. Powell WJ, DiBona DR, Flores J, Leaf A. The protective effect of hyperosmotic mannitol in myocardial ischemia and necrosis. *Circulation* 1976; 54: 603-15.

136. Fleetwood G, Poole-Wilson PA. Diastolic coronary resistance after ischaemia in the isolated rabbit heart: Effect of nifedipine. *J Mol Cell Cardiol* 1986; 18: 139-47.

137. Vogel WM, Cerel AW, Apstein CS. Post-ischaemic cardiac chamber stiffness and coronary vasomotion: The role of edema and effects of dextran. *J Mol Cell Cardiol* 1986; 18: 1207-18.

138. Humphrey SM, Thomson RW, Gavin JB. The influence of the no-reflow phenomenon on reperfusion and reoxygenation damage and enzyme release from ischemic isolated rat hearts. *J Mol Cell Cardiol* 1984; 16: 915-30.

139. Engler RL, Schmid-Schonbein GW, Pavalel RS. Leukocyte capillary plugging in myocardial ischaemia and reperfusion in the dog. *Am J Pathol* 1983; 111: 98-111.

140. Hearse DJ, Humphrey SM, Bullock GR. The oxygen paradox and the calcium paradox: Two facets of the same problem? *J Mol Cell Cardiol* 1978; 10: 641-68.

141. Hofmann M, Hofmann M, Genth K, Schaper W. The influence of reperfusion on infarct size after experimental coronary artery occlusion. *Basic Res Cardiol* 1980; 75: 572-82.

142. Jolly SR, Kane WJ, Bailie MB, Abrams GD, Lucchesi BR. Canine myocardial reperfusion injury: Its reduction by the combined administration of superoxide dismutase and catalase. *Circ Res* 1984; 54: 227-85.

143. Gaudel Y, Duvelleroy MA. Role of oxygen radicals in cardiac injury due to reoxygenation. *J Mol Cell Cardiol* 1984; 16: 459-70.

144. Ambrosio G, Weisfeldt ML, Jacobus WE, Flaherty JT. Evidence for a reversible radical-mediated component of reperfusion injury: Reduction by recombinant human superoxide dismutase administered at the time of reflow. *Circulation* 1987; 75: 282-91.

145. Olafson B, Forman MB, Puett DW, et al. Reduction of reperfusion injury in the canine preparation by intracoronary adenosine: Importance of the endothelium and the no-reflow phenomenon. *Circulation* 1987; 76: 1135-45.

146. Forman MB, Puett DW, Wilson BH, Vaughn WK, Friesinger GC, Virmani R. Beneficial long-term effect of intracoronary perfluorochemical on infarct size and ventricular function. *J Am Coll Cardiol* 1987; 9: 1082-90.

147. Kuroda H, Ishiguro S, Mori T. Optimal calcium concentration in the initial reperfusate for post-ischaemic myocardial performance (calcium concentration during reperfusion). *J Mol Cell Cardiol* 1986; 18: 625-33.

148. Shine KI, Douglas AM, Ricchiuti NV. Calcium, strontium, and barium movements during ischemia and reperfusion in rabbit ventricle. Implications for myocardial preservation. *Circ Res* 1978; 43: 712-20.

149. Shine KI, Douglas AM. Low calcium reperfusion of ischemic myocardium. *J Mol Cell Cardiol* 1983; 15: 252-60.

150. Stern MD, Chien AM, Capogrossi MC, Pelto DJ, Lakatta EG. Direct observation of the 'oxygen paradox' in single ventricular myocytes. *Circ Res* 1985; 56: 899-903.

151. Ferrari R, Ceconi C, Curello S, et al. Metabolic changes during post-ischaemic reperfusion. *J Mol Cell Cardiol* 1988; 20 (Suppl 2): 119-33.

152. Mauri F, De Biase AM, Franzosi MG, Pampallona S, Foresti A, Gasparini M. In-hospital cases of death in the patients admitted to the GISSI study. *G Ital Cardiol* 1987; 17: 37-44.

153. Poole-Wilson PA, Harding DP, Bourdillon PDV, Tones MA. Calcium out of control. *J Mol Cell Cardiol* 1984; 16: 175-87.

154. Marder VJ, Sherry S. Thrombolytic therapy: Current status. *N Engl J Med* 1988; 318: 1512-20, 1585-95.

155. Poole-Wilson PA. The nature of myocardial damage following reoxygenation. In: Parratt JR, ed. *Control and Manipulation of Calcium Movement.* New York: Raven Press, 1985: 325-40.

156. Jennings RB, Reimer KA. Lethal myocardial ischemic injury. *Am J Pathol* 1981; 102: 241-55.

157. Denton RM, McCormack JG. Calcium ions, hormones and mitochondrial metabolism. *Clin Sci* 1981; 61: 135-40.

158. Parr DR, Wimhurst JM, Harris EF. Calcium-induced damage of rat heart mitochondria. *Cardiovasc Res* 1975; 9: 366-72.

159. Murphy E, Aiton JF, Horres CR, Lieberman M. Calcium elevation in cultured heart cells: Its role in cell injury. *Am J Physiol* 1983; 245: C316

160. Wrogeman K, Pena SDJ. Mitochondrial calcium overload: A general mechanism for cell necrosis in muscle diseases. *Lancet* 1976; i: 672-4.

161. Shen AC, Jennings RB. Myocardial calcium and magnesium in acute ischemic myocardial injury. *Am J Pathol* 1972; 67: 417-40.

162. Shen AC, Jennings RB. Kinetics of calcium accumulation in acute myocardial ischemic injury. *Am J Pathol* 1972; 67: 441-52.

163. Bourdillon PD, Poole-Wilson PA. The effects of verapamil, quiescence and cardioplegia on calcium exchange and mechanical function in ischemic rabbit myocardium. *Circ Res* 1982; 50: 360-8.

164. Bourdillon PDV, Poole-Wilson PA. Effects of ischaemia and reperfusion on calcium exchange and mechanical function in isolated rabbit myocardium. *Cardiovasc Res* 1981; 15: 121-30.

165. Tones MA, Poole-Wilson PA. Alpha-adrenoceptor stimulation, lysophosphoglycerides, and lipid peroxidation in reoxygenation-induced calcium uptake in rabbit myocardium. *Cardiovasc Res* 1985; 19: 228-36.

166. Harding DP, Poole-Wilson PA. Calcium exchange in rabbit myocardium during and after hypoxia; effect of temperature and subtrate. *Cardiovasc Res* 1980; 14: 435-45.

167. Guarnieri T. Intracellular sodium-calcium dissociation in early contractile failure in hypoxic ferret papillary muscles. *J Physiol* 1987; 388: 449-65.

168. Allen DG, Orchard CH. Intracellular calcium concentration during hypoxia and metabolic inhibition in mammalian ventricular muscle. *J Physiol* 1983; 339: 107-22.

169. Cobbold PH, Bourne PK. Aequorin measurements of free calcium in single cells. *Nature* 1984; 312: 444-6.

170. Ganote CE, Kaltenbach JP. Oxygen-induced enzyme release: Early events and a proposed mechanism. *J Mol Cell Cardiol* 1979; 11: 389-406.

171. Jennings RB, Reimer KA, Steenbergen C. Myocardial ischaemia revisited. The osmolar load, membrane damage, and reperfusion. *J Mol Cell Cardiol* 1986; 18: 769-80.

172. Steenbergen C, Hill ML, Jennings RB. Volume regulation and plasma membrane injury in aerobic, anaerobic and ischemic myocardium in vitro: Effects of osmotic cell swelling on plasma membrane integrity. *Circ Res* 1985; 57(6): 864-75.

173. Burton KP, Hagler HK, Willerson JT, Buja LM. Abnormal lanthanum accumulation due to ischemia in isolated myocardium: Effect of chlorpromazine. *Am J Physiol* 1981; 10: H714-23.

174. Crake T, Poole-Wilson PA. Evidence that calcium influx on reoxygenation is not due to cell membrane disruption in the isolated rabbit heart. *J Mol Cell Cardiol* 1986; 18 (Suppl 4): 31-5.

175. Mak IT, Kramer JH, Weglicki WB. Potentiation of free radical-induced lipid peroxidation injury to sarcolemmal membranes by lipid amphophiles. *J Biol Chem* 1986; 261: 1153-7.

176. Lazdunski M, Frelin C, Vigne P. The sodium/hydrogen exchange system in cardiac cells: Its biochemical and pharmacological properties and its role in regulating internal concentrations of sodium and internal pH. *J Mol Cell Cardiol* 1985; 17: 1029-42.

177. Renlund DG, Gerstenblith G, Lakatta EG, Jacobus WE, Kallman CH, Weisfeldt ML. Perfusate sodium during ischaemia modifies post-ischaemic functional and metabolic recovery in the rabbit heart. *J Mol Cell Cardiol* 1984; 16: 795-801.

178. Grinwald PM. Calcium uptake during post-ischemic reperfusion in the isolated rat heart: Influence of extracellular sodium. *J Mol Cell Cardiol* 1982; 14: 359-65.

179. Poole-Wilson PA, Tones MA. Sodium exchange during hypoxia and on reoxygenation in the isolated rabbit heart. *J Mol Cell Cardiol* 1988; 20 (Suppl II): 15-22.

180. Allen DG, Orchard CH. Myocardial contractile function during ischemia and hypoxia. *Circ Res* 1987; 60: 153-68.

181. Kleber AG, Wilde AAM. Regulation of intracellular sodium ions in acute reversible myocardial ischemia: A perspective. *J Mol Cell Cardiol* 1986; 18 (Suppl 4): 27-30.

182. Whalen DA Jr, Hamilton DG, Ganote CE, Jennings RB. Effect of a transient period of ischemia on myocardial cells. I. Effects on cell volume regulation. *Am J Pathol* 1974; 74: 381-98.

183. Fiolet JWT, Baartscheer A, Schumacher CA, Coronel R, ter Welle HF. The change of free energy of ATP hydrolysis during global ischaemia and hypoxia in the rat heart. Its possible role in the regulation of transsarcolemmal sodium and potassium gradients. *J Mol Cell Cardiol* 1984; 16: 1023-36.

184. Steenbergen C, Hill ML, Jennings RB. Volume regulation and plasma membrane injury in aerobic, anaerobic and ischemic myocardium in vitro: Effects of osmotic cell swelling on plasma membrane integrity. Circ Res 1985; 57(6): 864-75.

185. Guarnieri C, Flamigni F, Calderera CM. Role of oxygen in the cellular damage induced by re-oxygenation of hypoxic heart. J Mol Cell Cardiol 1980; 12(8): 797-808.

186. Rao PS, Cohen MV, Mueller HS. Production of free radicals and peroxides in early experimental myocardial ischaemia. J Mol Cell Cardiol 1983; 15: 713-6.

187. Opie LH. Reperfusion injury and its pharmacologic modification. Circulation 1989; 80: 1049-62.

188. Engler R, Gilpin E. Can superoxide dismutase alter myocardial infarct size? Circulation 1989; 79: 1137-42.

189. Romson J, Hook B, Kunel S, Abrams G, Schork A, Lucchesi B. Reduction in the extent of ischemic myocardial injury by neutrophil depletion in the dog. Circulation 1983; 67: 1016-23.

190. Reimer KA, Jennings RB. Failure of the xanthine oxidase inhibitor allopurinol to limit infarct size after ischaemia and reperfusion in dogs. Circulation 1985; 71: 1069-75.

191. Loscalzo J, Braunwald E. Tissue plasminogen activator. N Engl J Med 1988; 319: 925-31.

192. Runge MS, Quertermous T, Haber E. Plasminogen activators: The old and the new. Circulation 1989; 79: 217-24.

193. DeWood MA, Spores J, Notske R, et al. Prevalence of total coronary occlusion during the early hours of transmural myocardial infarction. N Engl J Med 1980; 303: 897-902.

194. Dewood MA, Stifter WF, Simpson CS, et al. Coronary arteriographic findings soon after non-Q-wave myocardial infarction. N Engl J Med 1986; 315: 417-23.

195. Bush LR, Buja LM, Samowitz W, et al. Recovery of left ventricular segmental function after long-term reperfusion following temporary coronary occlusion in conscious dogs. Comparison of 2- and 4-hour occlusions. Circ Res 1983; 53: 248-63.

196. Lavallee M, Cox D, Patrick TA, Vatner SF. Salvage of myocardial function by coronary artery reperfusion 1, 2, and 3 hours after occlusion in conscious dogs. Circ Res 1983; 53: 235-47.

197. Reimer KA, Hill ML, Jennings RB. Prolonged depletion of ATP and of the adenine nucleotide pool due to delayed resynthesis of adenine nucleotides following reversible myocardial ischemic injury in dogs. J Mol Cell Cardiol 1981; 13: 229-39.

198. Hoffmeister HM, Mauser M, Schaper W. Repeated short periods of regional myocardial ischaemia: Effect on local function and high-energy phosphate levels. Basic Res Cardiol 1986; 81: 361-72.

199. Heyndrickx GR, Millard RW, McRitchie RJ, Maroko PR, Vatner SF. Regional myocardial functional and electrophysiological alterations after brief coronary artery occlusion in conscious dogs. J Clin Invest 1975; 56: 978-85.

200. Neely JR, Grotyohann LW. Role of glycolytic products in damage to ischemic myocardium. Dissociation of adenosine triphosphate levels and recovery of function of reperfused ischemic hearts. Circ Res 1984; 55: 816-24.

201. Murry CE, Jennings RB, Reimer KA. Preconditioning with ischaemia: A delay of lethal cell injury in ischemic myocardium. Circulation 1986; 74: 1124-36.

202. Rahimtoola SH. A perspective on the three large multicenter randomised clinical trials of coronary bypass surgery for chronic stable angina. Circulation 1985; 72 (Suppl 5): 123-35.

203. Jennings RB, Reimer KA, Hill ML, Mayer SE. Total ischemia in dog hearts, in vitro. Comparison of high-energy phosphate production, utilization, and depletion, and of adenine nucleotide catabolism in total ischemia in vitro vs severe ischemia in vivo. Circ Res 1981; 49: 892-900.

204. Swain JL, Sabina RL, McHale PA, Greenfield JC Jr, Holmes EW. Prolonged myocardial nucleotide depletion after brief ischemia in the open chest dog. Am J Physiol 1982; 242: H818-26.

205. Reimer KA, Lowe JE, Rasmussen MM, Jennings RB. The wavefront phenomenon of ischaemic cell death. 1. Myocardial infarct size vs duration of coronary occlusion in dogs. Circulation 1977; 56: 786-94.

206. Lowe JE, Cummings RG, Adams DH, Hull-Ryde EA. Evidence that ischemic cell death begins in the subendocardium independent of variations in collateral flow or wall tension. Circulation 1983; 68: 190-202.

207. Yellon DM, Hearse DJ, Crome R. Wyse RKH. Temporal and spatial characteristics of evolving cell injury during regional myocardial ischemia in the dog: The 'border zone' controversy. J Am Coll Cardiol 1983; 2: 661-70.

208. Poole-Wilson PA. Enzyme loss and calcium exchange in ischemic or hypoxic myocardium. In: Opie LH, ed. Calcium Antagonists and Cardiovascular Disease. New York: Raven Press, 1984: 97-104.

209. Kannel WB, Abbott RD. A prognostic comparison of asymptomatic left ventricular hypertrophy and unrecognized myocardial infarction: The Framingham Study. Am Heart J 1986; 111(2): 391-7.

210. Schang SJ, Pepine CJ. Transient asymptomatic ST-segment depression during daily activity. Am J Cardiol 1977; 39: 396-402.

211. Selwyn AP, Fox K, Eves M, Oakley D, Dargie H, Shillingford J. Myocardial ischaemia in patients with frequent angina pectoris. Br Med J 1978; 2: 1594-6.

212. Wood P. Da Costa's Syndrome (or Effort Syndrome). Br Med J 1941; 1: 767-72, 805-11.

213. White PD. The soldier's irritable heart: Certain observations of interest. JAMA 1942; 118: 270-1.

214. Herrick JB. Clinical features of sudden obstruction of the coronary arteries. JAMA 1912; 59: 2015-20.

215. Obrastzow WP, Straschenko ND. Zür Kenntis der Thrombose der Koronärarterien des Herzens. Z Klin Med 1910; 71: 116-25.

216. Epstein SE, Quyyumi AA, Bonow RO. Sudden death without warning. Possible mechanisms and implications for screening asymptomatic populations. N Engl J Med 1989; 321: 320-4.

217. Harris P. A theory concerning the course of events in angina and myocardial infarction. Eur J Cardiol 1975; 3: 157-63.

218. Mulcahy D, Keegan J, Crean P, et al. Silent myocardial ischaemia in chronic stable angina: A study of its frequency and characteristics in 150 patients. Br Heart J 1988; 60: 417-23.

219. Callaham PR, Froehlicher VF, Klein J, Risch M, Dubach P, Friis R. Exercise-induced silent ischemia: Age, diabetes, previous myocardial infarction and prognosis. J Am Coll Cardiol 1989; 14: 1175-80.

220. Knabb RM, Rosamond TL, Fox KA, Sobel BE, Bergmann SR. Enhancement of salvage of reperfused ischaemic myocardium by diltiazem. J Am Coll Cardiol 1986; 8: 861-71.

221. Kemp HG. Left ventricular function in patients with the anginal syndrome and normal coronary arteries. Am J Cardiol 1973; 32: 375-6.

222. Opherk D, Zebe H, Weihe E, et al. Reduced coronary dilatory capacity and ultrastructural changes of the myocardium in patients with angina pectoris but normal coronary angiograms. Circulation 1981; 63: 817-25.

223. Hutchison SJ, Poole-Wilson PA, Henderson AH. Angina with normal coronary arteries. Quart J Med 1989; New series 72, 268: 677-88.

224. Shapiro LM, Crake T, Poole-Wilson PA. Is altered cardiac sensation responsible for chest pain in patients with normal coronary arteries? Clinical observation during cardiac catheterisation. Br Med J 1988; 296: 170-1.

225. Cannon RO, Epstein SE. Microvascular angina as a cause of chest pain with angiographically normal coronary arteries. Am J Cardiol 1988; 61: 1338-43.

226. Cohn PF. Silent myocardial ischaemia: Review. Ann Intern Med 1988; 109: 312-7.

227. Mark DB, Hlatky MA, Califf RM, et al. Painless exercise ST deviation on the treadmill: Long-term prognosis. J Am Coll Cardiol 1989; 14: 885-92.

228. Ellestad MH, Savitz S, Bergdall D, Teske J. The false positive stress test. Multivariate analysis of 215 subjects with haemodynamic, angiographic and clinical data. *Am J Cardiol* 1977; 40: 681-5.

229. Froehlicher VF, Yanowitz FG, Thomas AS, Lacaster MC. The relation of coronary angiography and the electrocardiographic response to maximal treadmill testing in 76 asymptomatic men. *Circulation* 1973; 48: 597-604.

230. Mulcahy D, Keegan J, Sparrow J, Park A, Wright C, Fox K. Ischemia in the ambulatory setting – the total ischemic burden: Relation to exercise testing and investigative and therapeutic implications. *J Am Coll Cardiol* 1989; 14: 1166-72.

4
Arrhythmias Associated with Myocardial Ischaemia

Introduction

Coronary heart disease remains the most frequent cause of death in the Western world. Sudden cardiac death, defined as death within one hour of the onset of symptoms, accounts for between one-third and one-half of all such deaths (1,2). This represents approximately 20 deaths/million/week in most Western populations. Sudden cardiac death invariably reflects catastrophic collapse of the circulation, which may be caused by various cardiac events, such as myocardial rupture or left ventricular failure. However, cardiac arrest due to ventricular fibrillation is, by far, the most frequent cause and, while this may be the result of many forms of myocardial disease, acute myocardial ischaemia is most frequently the precipitating factor.

Approximately 50% of all deaths following within four weeks of an acute myocardial infarction occur during the first two hours post-infarction and, of these, over 80% are within the first hour (1). Patients at risk of developing ventricular fibrillation, therefore, have little time to seek medical aid (3) because of the brevity and perhaps surprisingly mild nature of the preceding symptoms. Thus, few victims of sudden cardiac death receive medical attention; for example, in one study, only 8% of patients dying within the first hour of a heart attack had been seen by a medical professional; this proportion falls to only 4.2% of those dying within the first 30 minutes (4).

Sudden cardiac death is sometimes observed in hospital, where successful resuscitation is most likely to be achieved. Most victims die outside of hospital where hospital-based medical practice has relatively little impact. Nevertheless, remarkable successes have been achieved through organized rapid delivery of medical care to patients threatened with impending myocardial infarction or death. A specially equipped and manned ambulance service was developed in Belfast, Northern Ireland, in 1966, which brought both a doctor and a defibrillator to patients threatened with acute myocardial infarction. This service allowed early resuscitation from ventricular fibrillation and brought early coronary care unit-type management to patients. The expense of providing this special ambulance service prompted other centres to integrate resuscitation schemes into existing emergency services, most notably in Seattle, Washington, in the US, and in Brighton, Sussex, in the UK (5,6). The success of these schemes is, to a considerable extent, dependent on local interest and enthusiasm, and may be more difficult to apply on a more widespread basis (7). Nevertheless, there is convincing evidence that community-based resuscitation facilities should be available in densely populated areas and at sites where large numbers of people gather, such as sports grounds, airports and railway stations.

The prevention of coronary disease is the method of choice for eradicating the clinical manifestations of coronary heart disease, including sudden cardiac death. For those with existing coronary disease and those for whom prevention remains elusive, ameliorating the effects of coronary disease is of considerable importance. Thus, reducing the frequency and severity of ischaemia, and attenuating its electrophysiological effects are essential in the management of these patients. This requires a detailed understanding of the mechanisms by which ischaemia disturbs the electrophysiological process which maintains normal sinus rhythm.

Regulation of normal sinus rhythm

Regularity of the cardiac rhythm is essential for coordination of the two mechanical properties of cardiac muscle, namely, contraction and relaxation. Maintenance of normal sinus rhythm and variation of the sinus rate depend principally on the integrity of the electrophysiological properties of the heart and on their responsiveness to autonomic and hormonal stimulation.

The electrophysiological properties of the heart may be summarized as:

Pacemaker activity;
Ordered conduction;
Refractoriness.

Arrhythmias may result from disorder of any one or more of these properties.

Pacemaker activity

In the normal heart, the pacemaker resides within the sinus node. The common electrophysiological property of all cells exhibiting pacemaker activity is diastolic depolarization. This causes the transmembrane potential to rise until the action-potential threshold is reached, at which point the next action potential is initiated (Figure 4.1). Pacemaker cells, therefore, have an intrinsic capacity to generate action potentials, unlike most cardiac myocytes which normally do not generate action potentials until the transmembrane potential is raised to the threshold value by the activity of adjacent cells (Figure 4.1).

Diastolic depolarization occurs in sinus node cells due to an inward current carried by sodium and calcium ions, and a reduced outward potassium current. This results in an increased intracellular positive charge, thus producing depolarization (8,9). Experimental studies may reveal pacemaker activity within other tissues, most notably the atrioventricular node and His-Purkinje fibres, but their rate of diastolic depolarization is normally slower than sinus node cells, with the result that each sinus beat causes depolarization before they attain the action-potential threshold (Figure 4.1). Thus, sinus node activity controls normal heart rhythm.

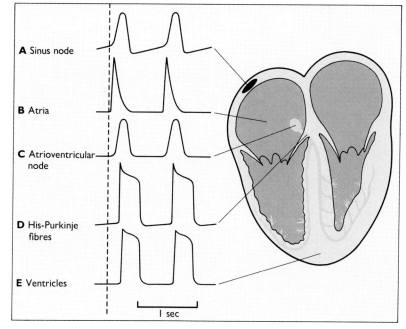

Figure 4.1 Cellular electrophysiology in different regions of the heart. Sinus and atrioventricular (AV) node action potentials have a slow upstroke velocity, thus accounting for the normal slow conduction properties of the AV node. Sinus node cells undergo gradual depolarization during diastole until the action-potential threshold is reached, at which time the next action potential is initiated. Atrial cells have shorter action potentials than ventricular cells, although they have a similar upstroke velocity. His-Purkinje cells have the fastest upstroke velocity (and fastest impulse propagation). By determining pacemaker activity, conduction velocity and duration of refractoriness, these electrophysiological properties regulate the cardiac rhythm.

Activity of the sinus node is mainly regulated by the autonomic nervous system; variation in heart rate in response to autonomic controls provides one of the most important mechanisms for altering cardiac output to meet changes in circulatory demands. Autonomic activity is centrally regulated in the brain stem, where information from higher cortical centres and peripheral sensors is integrated within the nucleus tractus solitarius (Figure 4.2) which, in turn, influences sympathetic outflow from the vasomotor centre, and parasympathetic outflow from the vagal nucleus. Parasympathetic preganglionic fibres leave the brain stem via the vagus nerve whereas sympathetic fibres radiate to intermediolateral columns in the spinal cord. Cardiac preganglionic sympathetic fibres arise from neurons in the intermediolateral columns of the upper eight thoracic segments and emerge in the rami communicantes of the upper six thoracic segments. Cardiac sympathetic fibres pass through the stellate ganglion, then via the ventral and dorsal ansa subclavia to join the vagal sympathetic trunk, forming a plexus of mixed nerves which innervate the heart.

Sympathetic fibres are distributed to the sinus node, atria, atrioventricular (AV) node, ventricles and coronary arteries;

Parasympathetic fibres pass to the sinus node, AV node, coronary arteries and, to a lesser extent, the atria (Figure 4.2).

Figure 4.2 Normal cardiac electrophysiology is regulated by autonomic nerve activity. Information from peripheral sensors and cortical areas is integrated in the tractus solitarius and influences parasympathetic output from the vagal nucleus and sympathetic output from the vasomotor centre. Parasympathetic fibres pass in the vagus nerve via the nodos ganglion; sympathetic fibres pass down the intermediolateral columns of the spinal cord and emerge through the upper 6-7 thoracic rami communicantes. These pass through the stellate ganglion and ansa subclavia to join the vagal parasympathetic fibres, forming the vagosympathetic trunk of mixed nerves which innervate the heart. Sinoatrial and atrioventricular node cells receive adrenergic and cholinergic fibres whereas ventricular myocardium receives predominantly adrenergic fibres.

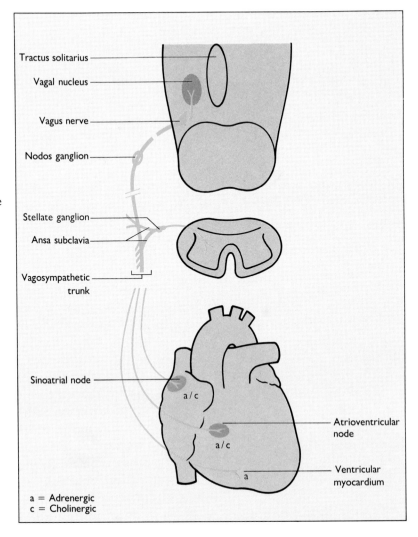

a = Adrenergic
c = Cholinergic

In the normal heart, autonomic activity regulates heart rate by changing the electrophysiological properties of sinus node cells (Figure 4.3). Sympathetic stimulation acts principally by increasing the rate of diastolic depolarization so that the action-potential threshold is reached earlier and heart rate is increased. Parasympathetic activity, on the other hand, causes the transmembrane potential to achieve more negative values in early diastole without changing the rate of diastolic depolarization so that a longer period is needed to reach the action-potential threshold (Figure 4.3, lower). By acting predominantly on pacemaker activity within the sinus node, chronotropic responses are normally restricted to the sinus node, which further acts to suppress abnormal pacemaker activity in other parts of the heart.

Figure 4.3 Electrophysiology of autonomic stimulation of sinus node cells. Sympathetic stimulation (upper) increases the slope of diastolic depolarization and thereby allows the action-potential threshold to be reached earlier, resulting in acceleration of the heart rate. Parasympathetic stimulation (lower) produces a more negative early diastolic potential so that, although the rate of diastolic depolarization is unchanged, a longer period is required to reach the action-potential threshold, resulting in a slower discharge rate.

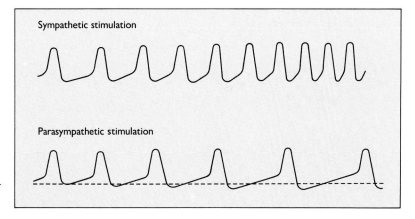

Sympathetic stimulation

Parasympathetic stimulation

Conduction

In addition to a properly functioning pacemaker, 'orderly' conduction is essential for maintenance of a regular rhythm. In the normal heart, the anatomical and physiological properties of the conducting system ensure than atrial and ventricular activation are well coordinated. Once the cardiac impulse has passed through the slow-conducting AV node, ventricular activation is rapid, normally complete in 120 msec due to the fast-conducting properties of the His-Purkinje fibres. While the slow-conducting properties of the AV node (approximately 5 mm/sec) act to protect the ventricles from rapid disorganized atrial activity, the His-Purkinje fibres ensure rapid coordinated ventricular activation (approximately 5 m/sec). Not only does this produce a uniform ventricular contraction, but also ensures synchronized depolarization and repolarization throughout the ventricles. Local areas of disordered conduction are a feature of many forms of myocardial disease, myocardial ischaemia in particular, and are of critical importance in the development of reentry arrhythmias.

Refractoriness

Once a normal cardiac myocyte has been depolarized, it cannot be depolarized again until a specific period of time, the so-called refractory period, has elapsed. In normal cells, although this corresponds closely with the action-potential duration, it varies depending on heart rate and may be altered by physiological factors which affect action-potential duration; in the normal human ventricle, it lasts for approximately 400 msec. This relatively long refractory period is a major difference between cardiac muscle and skeletal muscle, which has a refractory period of only a few milliseconds. It prevents cardiac muscle from becoming tetanized (unlike skeletal muscle) and ensures that contraction in cardiac muscle is rhythmic with an adequate period for ventricular filling, while also contributing to the orderly spread of activation through the heart. As a wave-front of depolarization is conducted through a segment of cardiac muscle, propagation can only proceed into areas as yet undepolarized, ensuring a forward progression of the wave front. This is important in preventing turning back or 'reentry' of activation into previously activated areas.

Electrophysiological disturbances which may lead to arrhythmias

Two circumstances may permit pacemaker activity outside the sinus node to become manifest and capture transiently or permanently the cardiac rhythm:

Pacemaker escape;
Acceleration of abnormal pacemakers.

Pacemaker escape

In the presence of complete heart block, the AV node fails to conduct sinus node impulses to the His-Purkinje system and ventricles. This allows a pacemaker within the ventricles to operate outside of sinus node control. Although the result is a regular rhythm of ±40 beats/minute, this rhythm is abnormal as it represents the 'escape' of a ventricular pacemaker from the suppressing influence of the sinus node. It may, in some circumstances, be life-saving by allowing ventricular contractions to continue.

Acceleration of pacemakers outside the sinus node

Acceleration of pacemaker activity may occur in ventricular or atrial myocardium for a number of reasons. As already discussed, sympathetic nerve stimulation increases the discharge frequency of the sinus node, and may also accelerate non-sinus node pacemakers. In the cat, for example, in the presence of sinus node suppression, stellate nerve stimulation increased idioventricular rate (10), a response which was abolished by beta-adrenergic blockade. The magnitude of this response, from 60 to 140 beats/minute, is not sufficient to escape sinus rhythm, which is normally approximately 180 beats/minute. Thus, uniform autonomic stimulation of the heart is not likely to produce an abnormal rhythm.

In contrast, non-uniform autonomic stimulation may be an important arrhythmogenic mechanism. During myocardial ischaemia, for example, there is convincing evidence that noradrenaline may be released into the ischaemic zone as a result of local pathophysiological conditions, such as high levels of extracellular potassium (see below). Such focal adrenergic stimulation may result in accelerated pacemaker activity locally, which may propagate into a ventricular arrhythmia. Experimental measurement of transmembrane potentials has demonstrated a number of mechanisms by which this may occur.

Increased automaticity

Increased automaticity: Accentuation of normal pacemaker activity.

As described above, neuronal beta-adrenergic stimulation increases the rate of diastolic depolarization in Purkinje fibres as well as in sinus node cells. When adrenergic stimulation is localized within ischaemic myocardium, it may increase automaticity locally without a concomitant increase in the sinus node rate, thus allowing the idioventricular rate to become the dominant cardiac rhythm. Such an idioventricular rhythm is often observed following acute myocardial infarction. It is slower than ventricular tachycardia, carries a relatively benign prognosis, and is the most frequent arrhythmia observed in association with successful reperfusion following coronary thrombolysis.

After-depolarizations

After-depolarizations: Oscillations in resting membrane potential following an action potential, so-called because they always follow an action potential and do not occur in isolation.

The importance of after-depolarizations is that they may result in attainment of the threshold potential; the additional action potentials thus induced may propagate through the heart, producing a tachycardia (11).

Two types of after-depolarizations are described:

Early after-depolarizations occur before complete repolarization of the preceding action potential, and in conditions of prolonged action-potential duration, whether induced by drugs such as quinidine, or by reduction of the repolarizing outward potassium current, as in hypokalaemia and at low heart rates.

Delayed after-depolarizations are oscillations following action-potential repolarization (11), and tend to arise in conditions leading to increased cell calcium content, such as digoxin toxicity, beta-adrenergic stimulation and high heart rates. Their importance lies in the possibility that oscillations in the transmembrane potential may reach threshold potential, thus generating repetitive action potentials and arrhythmias.

Investigation of after-depolarizations is based on the behaviour of single cells in response to a variety of toxic or pathological stimuli (11-13). The distinction made between after-depolarizations and pacemaker activity is based on their timing in relation to the preceding action potential and on the membrane potential at which they are initiated. Whether this represents fundamentally different mechanisms or only quantitative differences within the same process is not clear. It is possible that the observed differences in the arrhythmias associated with early and delayed after-depolarizations may simply reflect the different membrane potentials at which they are initiated. Indeed, both may best be considered mechanisms by which normally quiescent cells are induced into abnormal pacemaker activity.

Reentry

A reentry or circus-movement arrhythmia: Arrhythmia generated by a localized area of circular propagation from which secondary wave fronts are emitted to propagate throughout the heart.

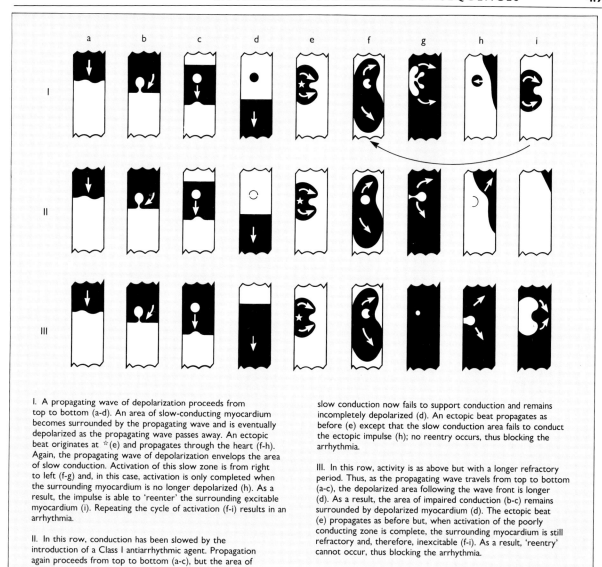

I. A propagating wave of depolarization proceeds from top to bottom (a-d). An area of slow-conducting myocardium becomes surrounded by the propagating wave and is eventually depolarized as the propagating wave passes away. An ectopic beat originates at ☆ (e) and propagates through the heart (f-h). Again, the propagating wave of depolarization envelops the area of slow conduction. Activation of this slow zone is from right to left (f-g) and, in this case, activation is only completed when the surrounding myocardium is no longer depolarized (h). As a result, the impulse is able to 'reenter' the surrounding excitable myocardium (i). Repeating the cycle of activation (f-i) results in an arrhythmia.

II. In this row, conduction has been slowed by the introduction of a Class I antiarrhythmic agent. Propagation again proceeds from top to bottom (a-c), but the area of slow conduction now fails to support conduction and remains incompletely depolarized (d). An ectopic beat propagates as before (e) except that the slow conduction area fails to conduct the ectopic impulse (h); no reentry occurs, thus blocking the arrhythmia.

III. In this row, activity is as above but with a longer refractory period. Thus, as the propagating wave travels from top to bottom (a-c), the depolarized area following the wave front is longer (d). As a result, the area of impaired conduction (b-c) remains surrounded by depolarized myocardium (d). The ectopic beat (e) propagates as before but, when activation of the poorly conducting zone is complete, the surrounding myocardium is still refractory and, therefore, inexcitable (f-i). As a result, 'reentry' cannot occur, thus blocking the arrhythmia.

Figure 4.4 Graphic illustration of how conduction and refractoriness influence reentry. The dark areas indicate depolarized and, therefore, refractory myocardium. Columns a-i illustrate sequential frames of activity; rows I-III represent activation sequences in three different circumstances. Disturbances in conduction and refractoriness are crucial for the development of arrhythmias. As shown here, the cardiac rhythm is dependent upon critical interaction between the rate of conduction and duration of refractoriness.

As already discussed, reactivation of previously depolarized tissue is normally prevented by refractoriness, which maintains an inexcitable barrier of tissue behind the propagating wave front (Figure 4.4, column a). This provides a safety margin of several hundred milliseconds in which small areas of non-uniform conduction may be resolved without leading to reentry. In some circumstances, conduction within a local area of disease may be so impaired that resolution may not be possible (Figure 4.4, columns b-d). Propagation through an area of poor conduction may be so disturbed that, by the time activation is completed, the surrounding myocardium is again excitable, thus permitting reentry of excitation (Figure 4.4, upper row).

In 1913, Mines (15) formulated the pathophysiological requirements for reentry:

An area of unidirectional block;
Impaired conduction;
Interruption of the reentry circuit abolishes the arrhythmia.

Two forms of reentry arrhythmias are encountered. In one, there is an 'anatomical' pathway, as in the various forms of preexcitation, for example, the Wolfe-Parkinson-White syndrome, which allows reactivation of the atria by waves propagated through the abnormal pathway from the ventricles. These are called macro-reentrant circuits as they involve a substantial amount of cardiac tissue.

The second type of reentrant circuit, the 'leading-circle model', is determined by electrophysiological disturbance within an area of myocardium. Essentially, circus activity propagates around an area of inexcitable tissue (16) from which wave fronts radiate centrifugally to produce a tachycardia.

In anatomically determined reentrant circuits, unlike the leading-circle model wherein path length is functionally determined by conduction velocity and refractoriness (16), the pathway is fixed in length and is usually large in comparison. In both types of reentry, whether or not there is activation of the reentry circuit is determined by conduction velocity and refractoriness; slow conduction and a shortened refractory period tend to increase the likelihood of reentry, and myocardial ischaemia produces both of these effects.

Arrhythmogenic mechanisms associated with myocardial ischaemia

Electrophysiological changes during ischaemia

Myocardial ischaemia produces rapid and profound changes in myocardial electrophysiology (Figure 4.5). A reduction in resting membrane potential lowers action-potential amplitude and upstroke velocity within minutes (17) (Figure 4.6) which, with continuing ischaemia, frequently spontaneously recovers (Figures 4.5 and 4.6).

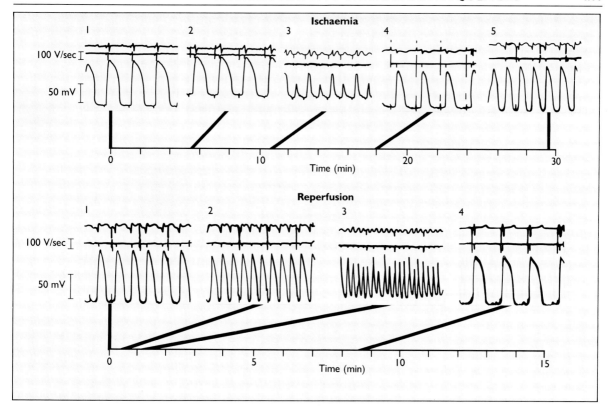

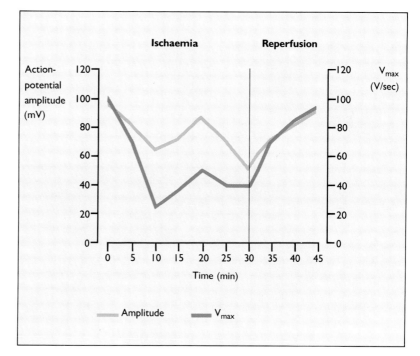

Figure 4.5 Cellular electrophysiological changes observed during myocardial ischaemia (upper) and reperfusion (lower). During ischaemia, action potentials become smaller and shorter and, in some cases, alternate action potentials are markedly reduced in amplitude and duration ('action potential alternans'; upper 3). During continued ischaemia, spontaneous electrophysiological recovery is frequently observed (upper 4 and 5). During reperfusion, electrophysiological recovery is rapid. In this case, ventricular tachycardia was present at the onset of reperfusion as action-potential amplitude and upstroke velocity recovered; the ventricular tachycardia accelerated (lower 2) before degenerating into ventricular fibrillation (lower 3).

Figure 4.6 Changes in action-potential amplitude and upstroke velocity (V_{max}) during ischaemia and reperfusion. Ischaemia causes a prompt fall in both, reaching a nadir at ± 10 minutes, after which spontaneous recovery is seen. Recovery commences promptly with reperfusion after 30 minutes of ischaemia and is complete in 15 minutes.

Measurement of refractory period during myocardial is-chaemia is difficult because stimulation thresholds change as ischaemia progresses. Using current clamp pulses and cir-cuitry permitting rapid change and measurement of stimulus strength, it has been possible to assess the refractory period at two-minute intervals during ischaemia. There is an initial pro-longation lasting approximately two to four minutes, followed by a shortening (17). Similar shortening occurs in action-poten-tial duration (Figure 4.7) although, at certain times, the nor-mally close correlation between refractory period and action-potential duration may be lost. Marked decreases in ampli-tude and duration of alternate action potentials (action poten-tial alternans; see Figure 4.5, upper 3) have been described as a transient phenomenon during experimental ischaemia, usu-ally lasting two to four minutes and often followed by par-tial spontaneous electrophysiological recovery (see Figures 4.5 and 4.6). Slowing of impulse conduction is expected during myocardial ischaemia as action-potential upstroke velocity is markedly reduced (17,18).

The distribution and uniformity of the electrophysiologi-cal changes taking place during ischaemia are important as-pects but difficult to measure. With millions of cells poten-tially involved in an area of ischaemia, it is inconceivable that transmembrane-potential measurements from one or even 10 cells can accurately reflect the patterns of change and distribu-tion. Similarly, measurement of conduction velocity between two points provides an average of a possible range of veloci-ties. There may, for example, be a small area of profoundly reduced conduction between the selected points which is by-passed by the propagating impulse. Such an area may have im-portant arrhythmogenic potential and yet have little effect on the measured conduction velocity.

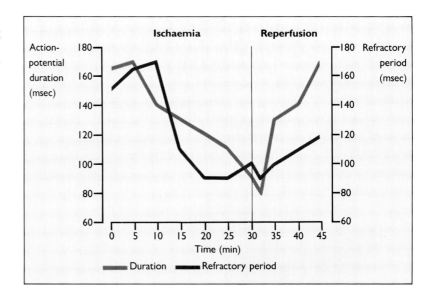

Figure 4.7 Changes in action-potential duration and refractory period during ischaemia and reperfusion. Following initial prolongation, ischaemia causes a reduction in both. Reperfusion causes a further transient, but significant, reduction in action-potential duration and refractory period. This precedes the onset of reperfusion arrhythmias and is followed by gradual recovery.

Electrophysiological measurements during ischaemia, therefore, only provide qualitative information concerning the direction of changes and serve as only a rough guide to their extent and distribution. Nevertheless, these provide important clues as to the possible arrhythmogenic mechanisms involved and potential antiarrhythmic interventions.

The time course of electrophysiological changes during ischaemia depends on many factors, including:

Severity of ischaemia at the site under study;
Extent of collateral development;
Metabolic demands of the tissue;
Heart rate;
Animal species.

Within individual models of ischaemia, distinct patterns of arrhythmias may be seen. Class IA and IB arrhythmias are said to occur between approximately two and 10 minutes, and 12 and 30 minutes, respectively, following coronary occlusion (19-21). This has led to the view that there may be two distinct arrhythmogenic mechanisms during ischaemia. However, a bimodal distribution of arrhythmias is not always observed and has not been clearly demonstrated in man, very likely a reflection of the variable rates of progress of ischaemia; for example, the sudden complete occlusion of a normal coronary artery, usually performed experimentally, is most unlikely to occur *in vivo*.

Attribution of particular mechanisms to arrhythmias on the basis of their observed time of occurrence following the onset of ischaemia may therefore be misleading.

Electrophysiological changes during reperfusion

For more than a century, it has been known that reperfusion of an area of ischaemic myocardium is capable of producing ventricular fibrillation (22).

Although most of our understanding of reperfusion arrhythmias is based on experimental studies, there is evidence that they also occur in man. Ventricular arrhythmias, for example, have been observed during the resolution of myocardial ischaemia and following coronary thrombolysis (23,24). However, although these observations do not indicate their frequency or clinical importance as a cause of sudden death, there is indirect evidence to suggest their involvement, and it is likely that reperfusion will continue to be studied as a potentially important arrhythmogenic mechanism.

The frequency of arrhythmias on reperfusion depends on the duration of the preceding ischaemic period. Reperfusion ventricular tachycardia and fibrillation are most likely to occur following 20 to 30 minutes of ischaemia, becoming less likely with shorter or longer episodes.

In the guinea-pig, reperfusion arrhythmias were not observed following ischaemia of less than five minutes' duration or of 60 minutes or longer. In contrast, following 30 minutes of ischaemia, reperfusion ventricular fibrillation occurred in 20/21 experiments (Figure 4.8). Thus, it appears that reperfusion arrhythmias require a critical amount of preceding myocardial damage; reperfusion is not arrhythmogenic if ischaemic damage is slight or if the myocardium is irreversibly damaged (17).

Reperfusion allows recovery from the electrophysiological changes provoked by the preceding period of ischaemia; action-potential amplitude and upstroke velocity both increase towards normal on reperfusion while action-potential duration and refractory period undergo further transient decreases prior to recovery (see Figure 4.7). The rate of recovery depends on the rate of reperfusion, with slower recovery and delayed onset of arrhythmias when reperfusion is gradual rather than

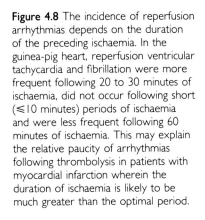

Figure 4.8 The incidence of reperfusion arrhythmias depends on the duration of the preceding ischaemia. In the guinea-pig heart, reperfusion ventricular tachycardia and fibrillation were more frequent following 20 to 30 minutes of ischaemia, did not occur following short (≤10 minutes) periods of ischaemia and were less frequent following 60 minutes of ischaemia. This may explain the relative paucity of arrhythmias following thrombolysis in patients with myocardial infarction wherein the duration of ischaemia is likely to be much greater than the optimal period.

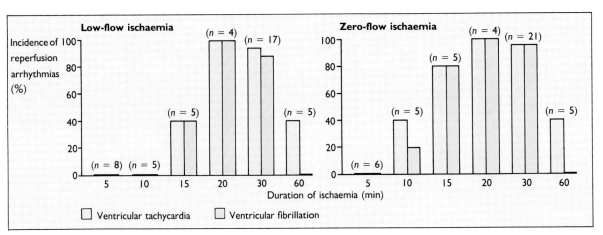

abrupt (Figure 4.9). The onset of reperfusion arrhythmias corresponds with early recovery and, in particular, with the transient reduction in refractory period which occurs in the first few minutes (see Figures 4.7 and 4.9). The tendency to develop reperfusion arrhythmias is usually short-lived. When reperfusion is abrupt, ventricular fibrillation commenced only rarely after five minutes and, following gradual reperfusion, it was rarely after six minutes (Figure 4.9).

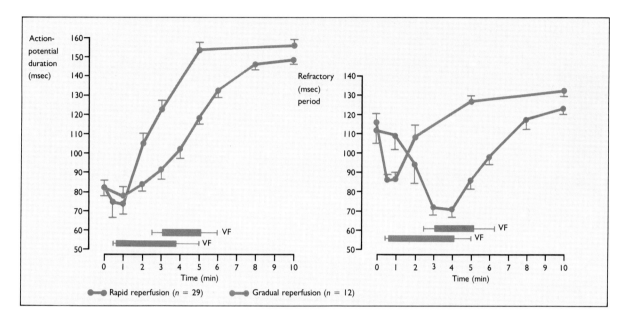

Figure 4.9 Changes in action-potential duration (left), refractory period (right), and onset and duration of ventricular fibrillation during gradual and rapid reperfusion. Transient reductions in action-potential duration and refractory period are observed in both groups, as is ventricular fibrillation (VF). Gradual reperfusion delays the onset of VF and slows the electrophysiological changes. However, in both cases, reduction in action-potential duration and refractory period precedes the onset of arrhythmias, indicating that these changes are likely to be important in mediating the arrhythmogenic effects of reperfusion.

In order to identify electrophysiological changes associated with reperfusion arrhythmias, electrophysiological responses to reperfusion following brief (five minutes) and prolonged (60 minutes) periods of ischaemia (when arrhythmias are uncommon) were compared with those following 30 minutes of ischaemia (when ventricular tachycardia and fibrillation are at maximum). In general, following short ischaemic periods, action potentials were least altered, and recovery was most rapid and complete on reperfusion.

In contrast, reperfusion following prolonged ischaemia produced more gradual recovery which was less complete. Reperfusion after 30 minutes of ischaemia produced prompt recovery in action potentials but, in the case of action-potential duration, further transient reduction preceded recovery. This feature was observed almost immediately on reperfusion, before the onset of arrhythmias, and was not observed with reperfusion following five or 60 minutes of ischaemia, but was maximum at approximately 60 to 90 seconds of reperfusion, corresponding with the onset of arrhythmias (17). This combination of reducing action-potential duration and refractoriness at a time when upstroke velocity (and consequently conduction) are improving is very likely to render the heart vulnerable to arrhythmias. Furthermore, conditions in which arrhythmias are inhibited during reperfusion, such as brief or prolonged periods of preceding ischaemia, alpha-adrenoceptor blockade or catecholamine depletion, also appear to inhibit transient reduction in action-potential duration (25,26).

Interaction between delayed conduction and altered refractoriness

Vulnerability to arrhythmias reflects disturbances in automaticity, conduction and/or refractoriness (see above) which occur soon after the onset of ischaemia and for a considerable time during reperfusion; yet, arrhythmias occur within relatively limited periods. The most likely explanation is that the degree of vulnerability to arrhythmias is related not only to the extent of disturbance but also to the relative changes in conduction and refractoriness, and their distribution.

After prolonged ischaemia, electrophysiological changes may be so marked that conduction and activation cannot be sustained sufficiently to allow the propagation of arrhythmias. Similarly, at the onset of ischaemia, some time is required for the electrophysiological changes to reach arrhythmogenic potential. During reperfusion, arrhythmias arise much earlier than during ischaemia, very likely a reflection of the much more rapid rate of electrophysiological changes during reperfusion.

There is no absolute threshold value of automaticity, conduction or refractoriness beyond which arrhythmias become inevitable; rather, it appears that disturbances of electrophysiology increase myocardial vulnerability to arrhythmias. These are:

Increased automaticity;
Delayed conduction;
Reduced or variable refractoriness.

The extent of change required in any one mechanism to produce arrhythmias depends on the state of the others; for example, a minor delay in conduction may be sufficient in the presence of markedly reduced and variable refractoriness. Similarly, increased automaticity may produce ectopic beats of little clinical significance in the presence of normal conduction and refractoriness, yet prove lethal by initiating ventricular fibrillation if conduction and refractoriness are disturbed, as with myocardial ischaemia. However, markedly delayed conduction may in fact inhibit the development of arrhythmias by impairing their propagation and is the most likely explanation for the natural attenuation of arrhythmias following the early stages of acute myocardial infarction.

Other factors which influence the vulnerability to arrhythmias are:

The amount of ischaemic myocardium;
The degree of variability between adjacent areas.

Clearly, the extent, variability and distribution of electrophysiological changes during ischaemia can only be described in approximate terms at present, particularly in acute infarction, when information is limited to surface electrocardiography (ECG). Although designing interventions based on a complete understanding of the pathophysiology of a particular case is not possible, despite this limitation, considerable progress has been made towards understanding the underlying mechanisms and their modification.

Late arrhythmias following infarction
Once the initial phase of acute myocardial infarction is over, the tendency to develop arrhythmias usually diminishes dramatically, although there is a continued risk of sudden cardiac death in the subsequent months.

Most patients who die suddenly from coronary heart disease have had previous myocardial infarction (27), and almost all of those with sustained ventricular tachycardia have had previous infarctions. The mechanisms which may be contributory include:

Postinfarction ischaemia;
Incomplete infarction;
Reocclusion following recanalization;
Ventricular aneurysm.

Postinfarction ischaemia
Patients with postinfarction ischaemia may have extensive coronary disease affecting myocardial blood supply not involved in the infarct (27), rendering them susceptible to ischaemia or infarction in new areas of myocardium. Such episodes certainly present further periods in which the heart is

vulnerable to arrhythmias and, indeed, experimental studies suggest that acute ischaemia in the presence of existing healed infarction may be especially dangerous as electrophysiological uniformity is more disturbed. Acute ischaemia in these hearts may reduce refractoriness in the acute infarct zone and prolong refractoriness in the healed infarct zone while having no effect on uninvolved tissue (27).

> Myocardial infarction is an important risk factor for sudden cardiac death because:
>
> It is an obvious marker of severe coronary disease;
> Healed infarction may increase the arrhythmogenic risks associated with a second infarct.

Incomplete infarction

Early studies of healed myocardial infarction revealed little evidence of continued electrophysiological instability (28,29), apparently due to extensive necrosis in the infarct zone leading to electrophysiological extinction. Furthermore, in later studies, infarcts with less extensive necrosis and survival of some ischaemic tissue exhibited persistent arrhythmogenic potential (30-32). The distribution of necrosis is less uniform in these infarcts, and scar tissue is formed between bands of surviving myocardium with a greater potential for electrophysiological variability. In particular, cells at boundaries between normal and scar tissue may show non-uniform electrophysiology and respond well to drugs or sympathetic nerve stimulation.

Reocclusion following recanalization

The extent of necrosis following coronary occlusion depends on the size and position of the artery involved, the extent of collateral vessel supply to the ischaemic area and the duration of coronary occlusion. In cases where recanalization is early, although more myocardium survives, this tissue is dependent on an unreliable blood supply. Reocclusion may occur with further risk of developing arrhythmias.

Ventricular aneurysm

In hearts with large myocardial infarction, the ventricular wall may be so weakened that it stretches during systole, producing what is described clinically as a ventricular aneurysm, which has a recognized high risk of developing persistent ventricular arrhythmias. All of the mechanisms already described may be applicable. In addition, systolic stretching of cells at the boundary between normal myocardium and the aneurysm may produce depolarization with the attendant risks of increased automaticity and altered conduction. Mapping studies carried out in patients during surgery have shown that arrhythmias tend to arise from areas bordering on the aneurysm rather than within the aneurysm itself (33). Resection of the involved myocardium may be effective in suppressing these arrhythmias, and is best carried out in conjunction with mapping techniques to delineate the arrhythmogenic focus (34).

Previous myocardial infarction is a risk factor for sudden cardiac death because it defines patients with significant coronary disease and results in areas of myocardium with permanently disturbed electrophysiology. Recognition of patients at greatest risk rests on:

Detection of myocardium with jeopardized coronary supply beyond the infarct zone;
Recognition of patients with severe left ventricular dysfunction.

Mechanisms underlying electro-physiological changes during ischaemia

As already stated, all arrhythmias reflect disturbances of the normal electrophysiological control mechanisms: Conduction; refractoriness; automaticity. In order to understand how these change during ischaemia and, perhaps more importantly, how these changes may be prevented, it is essential to investigate the causal mechanism. Recently, this has received considerable attention and several important factors have been identified.

Adrenergic influences

There is strong clinical and experimental evidence that adrenergic activity is increased in acute myocardial ischaemia and infarction (35,36).

Plasma and urinary catecholamine levels are increased following acute myocardial infarction (37,38).

Experimental myocardial ischaemia *in vivo* or in isolated hearts has shown loss of myocardial noradrenaline (35,39,40).

These findings indicate that infarction causes adrenergic activation which appears to be selectively greater in ischaemic myocardium.

Indirect evidence that the release of catecholamines contributes to the arrhythmogenic process is provided by experiments in which myocardial denervation by chemical (10,26,41) or surgical (42,43) techniques has reduced the incidence of arrhythmias during ischaemia. Treatment of cats or guinea-pigs with 6-hydroxydopamine reduces myocardial noradrenaline to approximately 5% of the level in controls (10,26), and significantly reduces ventricular tachycardia and fibrillation during ischaemia and reperfusion. Similar results have been reported with surgical denervation, but Ebert and colleagues (42) concluded that, as denervation was not effective if carried out immediately prior to coronary ligation, the response to denervation must be dependent on myocardial catecholamine depletion, which takes several days.

Studies based on adrenoceptor blockade provide further evidence of adrenergic involvement in the arrhythmogenic process. Many studies have investigated the effect of beta-adrenoceptor blockade (for review, see 49) during ischaemia and, although some protection is generally observed, the results are more variable than with denervation. This may be a reflection of several factors such as:

1 Inadequate drug levels within the ischaemic area;
2 Overwhelming local catecholamine release at a critical period during the ischaemic process;
3 Altered tissue sensitivity to adrenergic stimulation during ischaemia.

In addition, there is sound evidence that beta-adrenoceptor blockade reduces the risk of sudden cardiac death following acute myocardial infarction (45,46). More recently, alpha-adrenoceptor blockade has been shown to reduce the incidence of ventricular arrhythmias during experimental ischaemia and reperfusion (10,25,47).

Although there is evidence that catecholamine release is important during ischaemia and reperfusion, the mechanism of release is unclear. There is evidence that neural activity is increased during early ischaemia (43) concomitant with the development of arrhythmias, but whether this is primarily or in part responsible for catecholamine release during ischaemia is less well-defined. Ischaemia in isolated perfused hearts (and therefore devoid of neural connexions) has been shown to cause catecholamine release (39,40). Catecholamine release is greater in ischaemic tissue than in adjacent normal myocardium (48). Surgical denervation is more effective when carried out well before coronary ligation when depletion would have occurred (42).

Thus, the evidence suggests that local changes within the ischaemic myocardium play an important role in promoting catecholamine release. Nevertheless, there is convincing evidence that artificially generated stress conditions increase the arrhythmogenic effects of acute myocardial ischaemia (49), which correlates with increased levels of circulating catecholamines. In a study with dogs in which stress was induced by denying access to food, their heart rates and blood pressure were increased and they were three times more likely to develop ventricular fibrillation during ischaemia and reperfusion than non-stressed animals (49).

Thus, increased adrenergic activity appears to play a major role in producing acute ischaemia, and the level of autonomic nerve activity has an important influence. However, the extent to which the anxiety and alarm experienced during acute myocardial infarction contributes to the development of arrhythmias is difficult to determine.

The past decade has seen considerable interest in the possible role of alpha-adrenoceptor stimulation in the genesis of arrhythmias during ischaemia and reperfusion. Several alpha-blocking drugs have been shown to reduce the incidence of ventricular fibrillation in the cat (10), dog (47) and guinea-pig (25) during ischaemia and reperfusion. The most important associated electrophysiological action is attenuation of the ischaemia-induced reductions in action-potential duration and refractory period (25). Similar changes were observed in hearts depleted of catecholamines (26) and, more importantly, were reversed by perfusion with the alpha-agonist methoxamine. Furthermore, methoxamine reversed the antiarrhythmic effect of catecholamine depletion, thus increasing the incidence of ventricular tachycardia and fibrillation (Figure 4.10). Exogenous adrenoceptor stimulation is arrhythmogenic during ischaemia and reperfusion, and alpha-blockade is one of the most powerful means of inhibiting the development of arrhythmias, whereas alpha-adrenoceptor stimulation of normal myocardium produces only minor effects, namely, prolongation in action-potential duration and a weak positive inotropism (36). The much greater changes observed during ischaemia suggest that myocardial sensitivity to alpha-adrenoceptor activity is altered by the ischaemia.

Thus, although alpha-adrenoceptor stimulation during ischaemia induces ventricular tachycardia and fibrillation, it is not arrhythmogenic during normal perfusion (50); similarly, intracoronary infusion of methoxamine in the cat had no effect on idioventricular rate during normal perfusion, but

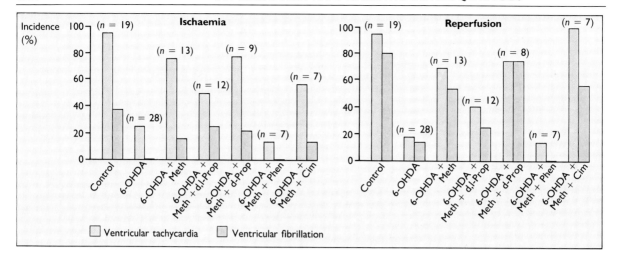

Figure 4.10 Incidence of ventricular tachycardia (VT) and fibrillation (VF) during ischaemia and reperfusion in isolated perfused guinea-pig hearts. Myocardial catecholamine depletion with 6-hydroxydopamine (6-OHDA) reduces the incidence of VT and VF during ischaemia and reperfusion. Although perfusion of similarly treated hearts with the alpha-adrenoceptor agonist methoxamine (Meth) increases the incidence of VT and VF, indicating its arrhythmogenic potential, this effect was abolished by the alpha-blocker phentolamine (Phen), but not by propranolol (Prop) or H_2-receptor blockade with cimetidine (Cim). These findings support the concept that local myocardial catecholamines are involved in the arrhythmogenic effects of ischaemia and reperfusion, and that these effects are mediated in part by alpha-adrenoceptor stimulation.

caused marked acceleration during early reperfusion (10). A reversible increase in the number of alpha-adrenoceptors during ischaemia has been observed in the cat (51), but not in the rat (52) or guinea-pig (53). The mechanism of increased myocardial sensitivity to alpha-agonists during ischaemia therefore remains unresolved. These findings have not been tested in man as most available alpha-blockers also act at peripheral sites in the circulation, thus causing vasodilatation which may lead to hypotension and reduced coronary perfusion. However, the availability of new compounds with cardioselective properties (54) should allow useful clinical trials to be undertaken in future.

Effects of increased extracellular potassium

The ratio of intracellular to extracellular potassium is one of the determinants of resting membrane potential, and the observation that ischaemic cells leak potassium ions was readily recognized as a possible basis of the electrophysiological changes and arrhythmias during myocardial ischaemia (55-57). Early attempts to assess potassium release were based on measurements of arteriovenous differences, but this proved to be inadequate as much released potassium accumulates because of poor tissue perfusion.

The development of ion-sensitive electrodes has permitted useful measurements to be obtained of the rate and extent of potassium accumulation in the extracellular space of ischaemic tissue (for reviews, see 58 and 59). Using this technique, extracellular potassium has been shown to rise 15 seconds following coronary occlusion in the pig, reaching levels of approximately 12 to 15 mmol/l at 10 minutes (58,59). During the next 20 to 30 minutes, the rate of accumulation was slower, but gradually increased again, thereafter reaching levels of 20 to 30 mmol/l at 60 minutes (Figure 4.11). The severity of ischaemia depends on the size of vessel occluded although, within a single infarct,

Figure 4.11 Measurements of extracellular potassium using ion-selective electrodes demonstrate rapid elevation (within 15 seconds) following the onset of ischaemia. Following an initial rise to ±12 mmol/l, the rate of accumulation decreases until ±20 minutes, after which the levels rise more steeply again. (After **Gettes, 1987**)

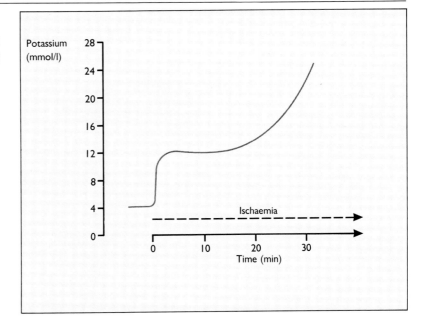

variations in the severity of ischaemia and its associated pathophysiology have been observed (60). There is a gradation of ischaemic effects between normal tissue and the centre of the ischaemic zone, including varying degrees of potassium accumulation (59), which is very likely to produce further regional variations in cardiac electrophysiology during ischaemia, thus adding to the susceptibility to arrhythmias.

The extent of the observed increases in extracellular potassium are certainly sufficient to produce marked electrophysiological changes, namely, reduced resting membrane potential, action-potential amplitude, and upstroke velocity and duration with delayed conduction. As similar changes are observed during ischaemia, the reported elevations in extracellular potassium must contribute to the electrophysiological changes associated with ischaemia. However, it is more difficult to determine the extent to which the electrophysiological changes are due solely to the accumulation of potassium.

Hill and Gettes (61) demonstrated spontaneous electrophysiological recovery between five and 20 minutes following coronary ligation, when potassium accumulation was increasing rapidly. Attempts have been made to correlate potassium accumulation with the development of arrhythmias, in particular, the early rapid rise in potassium may be related to the early phase Class IA arrhythmias and the later rise with Class IB arrhythmias. Such associations should, however, be regarded as only temporal. Further work is needed to prove causality between the timing of potassium accumulation and ventricular fibrillation.

Oxygen-derived free radicals

Free radicals are molecules with one unpaired electron in an outer orbital. They are intensely reactive chemically, making them toxic to tissues, and attract electrons from a wide variety of molecules, thereby producing new free radicals in a chain reaction. The absence of oxygen during myocardial ischaemia contributes to the formation of a wide variety of reduced metabolites which accumulate, thus providing a large pool of available electrons. Reappearance of oxygen during subsequent reperfusion may then lead to oxidation and free radical formation by several reactions (62).

At present, evidence that free-radical production may contribute to the development of arrhythmias, especially during reperfusion, is indirect:

Interventions which should reduce free-radical formation have been shown to exert antiarrhythmic effects;

Conversely, stimulation of radical production has been found to be arrhythmogenic (63).

Further work is needed to clarify this issue.

Platelets

Platelets are a potentially rich source of vasoactive substances, such as serotonin and thromboxane A_2. Their release during ischaemia may exacerbate the severity and extent of necrosis.

There is evidence that platelets:

May aggravate ischaemia when infused directly into isolated perfused hearts (64);

When depleted using platelet antiserum, reduce the frequency of arrhythmias (65) and extent of necrosis (65,66) during ischaemia.

Their deposition at sites of arterial wall injury may lead to vasospasm and further reduce blood flow (67).

The main focus of work at present is investigation of the mechanisms leading to platelet activation and distinguishing the mediators of tissue damage. A phospholipid with highly potent effects on platelets (PAF; platelet activating factor) may be important in initiating and perpetuating platelet activation. However, further work is needed to clarify whether the aggravation of ischaemia is due to direct myocardial effects of substances released from platelets or indirect effects of vasoconstriction.

Arrhythmias associated with acute myocardial infarction

Acute myocardial infarction may produce any form of arrhythmia, ventricular arrhythmias being the most frequent and most serious. As already described, ventricular arrhythmias following experimental ischaemia often arise only within particular periods of time. Acute myocardial infarction, however, is variable in its rate of onset which, in turn, determines the period of vulnerability to arrhythmias. The evolution of Q waves is the most striking clinical indicator of evolving myocardial infarction, and may take place in as little time as 30 minutes (Figure 4.12), or be protracted over several hours. In addition, the development of Q waves may be preceded by one or more episodes of transient ischaemia that may be severe and capable of producing marked changes on ECG, usually in the form of an ST-segment elevation which resolves completely at the end of the ischaemic episode (Figure 4.13).

Alternans of the ST segment is an unusual, but well described, finding on ECG during the evolution of acute myocardial infarction, and may be restricted to only one lead and may be transient. The example shown in Figure 4.14 appeared 12 minutes after the onset of chest pain and lasted for just over three minutes. The cellular electrophysiological counterpart of ST-segment alternans (see Figure 4.5) is when alternate action potentials are reduced in amplitude and duration. These ECG changes reflect the variable rates of thrombotic occlusion (discussed in depth in another section). The timing of ventricular fibrillation following the onset of infarction usually cannot be determined as accurately in man as in experimental models of ischaemia, but it is nevertheless clear that ventricular fibrillation is most likely to occur soon after the onset of ischaemia. The patient whose ECG is shown in Figure 4.12 developed ventricular fibrillation 14 minutes after the onset of chest pain and before Q waves had completely evolved. This early occurrence of ventricular fibrillation explains why approximately half of all deaths during the first four weeks of infarction occur within the first two hours, and why so many victims of sudden cardiac death fail to reach medical attention.

Figure 4.12 Successive ECG recordings (lead V2) taken during the development of acute anteroseptal myocardial infarction. The times indicate the interval following the onset of chest pain. Initially, there is marked ST-segment elevation with Q waves already present at eight minutes following the onset of pain. Thereafter, Q waves deepen as the ST-segment elevation regresses. Ectopic beats were recorded at 12 minutes and ventricular fibrillation at 15 minutes.

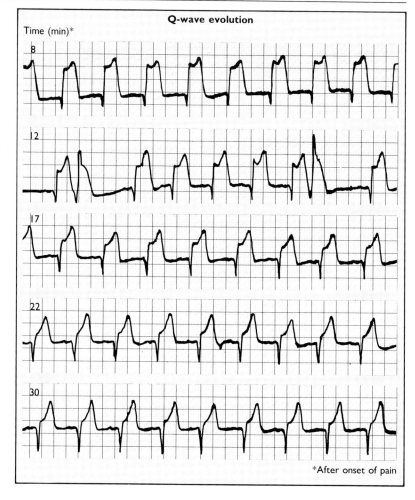

Ventricular fibrillation

Ventricular fibrillation is the most important complication of acute myocardial infarction because of its frequency, lethality and treatability, circumstances permitting. It is easily recognized on ECG as rapid, irregular and disorganized ventricular activity.

Ventricular fibrillation is said to be primary when it occurs early following the onset of infarction in the absence of shock or heart failure, in contradistinction from late (secondary) fibrillation in patients with cardiogenic shock or fibrillation. Both designations may be misleading as both are caused by myocardial ischaemia; there is little evidence to indicate that secondary ventricular fibrillation is a complication of cardiac failure or shock rather than the underlying myocardial ischaemia. Nevertheless, there are important differences between the two types.

Figure 4.13 Twelve-lead ECG recorded during an episode of severe chest pain with unstable angina. Elevation of the ST segment is present in all of the chest leads and most marked in V2 to V4. This episode of pain lasted for 15 minutes, and the ECG changes were completely resolved by 20 minutes after the onset of pain. Such changes indicate that transient ischaemia may cause profound electrophysiological changes. Experimental evidence suggests that such episodes may be capable of leading to serious arrhythmias, including ventricular fibrillation.

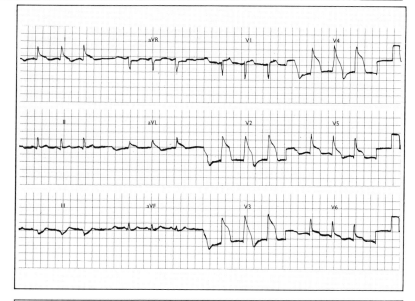

Figure 4.14 ST-segment alternans: Alteration in the degree of ST-segment elevation between successive beats. In this case (same patient as in Figure 4.12), this was observed at 14 minutes following the onset of chest pain. Observation was for a period of three minutes and was limited to one ECG lead only. The most likely explanation of this appearance is action-potential alternans (see Figure 4.5, upper 3).

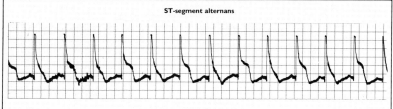

ST-segment alternans

Primary ventricular fibrillation

The incidence of primary ventricular fibrillation falls sharply soon after the onset of infarction, and the infarct size has only a small effect on its frequency. It was thought that the frequency of ectopic beats might predict the likelihood of its occurrence (68,69), but this has not been substantiated by further studies (70). Treatment of ventricular fibrillation by immediate direct-current (DC) cardioversion where possible is highly successful in almost all cases; if carried out promptly, the ventricular fibrillation has little effect on the prognosis (71). Nevertheless, these patients are at risk of further episodes of ventricular fibrillation and should therefore be monitored in a coronary care unit for 24 to 48 hours whether prophylactic antiarrhythmic treatment is given or not.

There is sound evidence that prophylactic treatment with lignocaine can reduce the incidence of ventricular fibrillation (72), but the dose required is high and side-effects are common. For patients in efficient coronary care units where ventricular fibrillation can be detected and cardioverted promptly, prophylactic antiarrhythmic treatment is usually not necessary, whereas patients seen outside of hospital with little prospect of being admitted to hospital promptly should receive prophylactic treatment.

Secondary ventricular fibrillation

Extensive myocardial infarction with cardiac failure or shock carries a poor prognosis; many of these patients die from ventricular fibrillation. Cardioversion is frequently unsuccessful and antiarrhythmic treatment disappointing. Approximately half of those who are resuscitated will die during the following year (73). Treatment is aimed at achieving meticulous control of recurrent ischaemia and optimal treatment of heart failure. Patients who also have other ventricular arrhythmias, such as couplets, frequent multifocal ectopics or tachycardia, should be given antiarrhythmic treatment. Some of these patients will be found to have ventricular aneurysms and, if unresponsive to medical treatment, should be considered for aneurysmectomy with intraoperative mapping to ensure that excision includes important areas of electrical instability.

Ventricular tachycardia

> **Ventricular tachycardia** is defined as three or more consecutive ventricular ectopic beats occurring at a rate of more than 120/minute. Brief runs of ventricular tachycardia (three to 10 beats) are common in the early phase of acute infarction and do not appear to carry an adverse prognosis.

Sustained ventricular tachycardia usually arises in the later stages of infarction and may present after discharge from hospital. Its haemodynamic consequences are somewhat variable; some patients are barely aware of it while others are profoundly shocked during an episode. There is always a possibility that sustained ventricular tachycardia may degenerate into fibrillation, particularly if there is concomitant hypotension. For this reason, ventricular tachycardia should be treated promptly, by DC cardioversion for patients with hypotension or shock, and medical treatment for those who are not compromised. Establishing effective preventive treatment is important and may be assisted by invasive electrophysiological testing. However, it is essential to ascertain, by ECG telemetry or ambulatory monitoring, that the treatment does prevent the occurrence of spontaneous attacks. Sustained ventricular tachycardia is a well recognized complication of ventricular aneurysm, and surgery may be helpful for patients who fail to respond to medical treatment.

Reperfusion arrhythmias

As already discussed, there is sound evidence that reperfusion of ischaemic myocardium may cause ventricular arrhythmias (23-25). Coronary thrombolysis for achieving coronary recanalization in acute infarction is of proven benefit in preserving myocardial function and reducing mortality. Experience so far has demonstrated that reperfusion associated with thrombolysis may lead to arrhythmias, including ventricular fibrillation but, in practice, serious arrhythmias are uncommon.

In this author's experience, the most frequent rhythm disturbance is an idioventricular rhythm with a rate of 90 to 110/minute. Haemodynamic embarrassment is unusual and sinus rhythm is usually spontaneously restored. The relative scarcity of ventricular tachycardia and fibrillation following thrombolysis in comparison to experimental reperfusion is best explained by the relatively long interval between the onset of chest pain and reperfusion, which is further supported by experimental studies in which reperfusion at 60 minutes or more after the onset of ischaemia caused few arrhythmias (17). Few patients receive thrombolytic therapy within 60 minutes, and recanalization and reperfusion may take a further 30 to 60 minutes.

> There is clear evidence that the efficacy of thrombolysis is related to how soon it is begun, which should lead its earlier administration; in this event, experimental evidence predicts that reperfusion arrhythmias will become more frequent.

> The introduction of thrombolytic therapy in the very early stages of acute infarction out of hospital should be carried out with caution until further experience is available.

Areas for future development

The magnitude of the problem of sudden death due to ventricular arrhythmias and the fact that it remains substantially unaltered by medical treatment indicates the need for continued research in this area. The antiarrhythmic drugs currently available are characterized by their effects on normal cardiac electrophysiology, which may be helpful in predicting their efficacy for particular arrhythmias, for example, calcium antagonists for supraventricular tachycardia, and beta-blockers for exercise- or stress-related arrhythmias. It is less useful in the context of myocardial ischaemia in which cardiac electrophysiology is severely disturbed and the effects of the drug are minor in comparison.

Work is needed to develop compounds which act specifically on ischaemic myocardium to reduce the effects of ischaemia and reperfusion. These compounds may have little or no direct action on 'normal' cardiac electrophysiology, but may act at several intra- and extracellular sites to reduce or retard the progress of ischaemia. This work will require a shift away from the traditional methods of assessing antiarrhythmic actions towards greater emphasis on modifications of the electrophysiology accompanying ischaemia.

A number of potentially important mechanisms have been identified as possible mediators of the arrhythmogenic effects of ischaemia:

Alpha-adrenergic activity, free-radical production and platelet activity are most likely to be productive.

Further research is needed to develop these possibilities to ultimately test their applicabiity to man.

References

1. Armstrong A, Duncan B, Oliver MF, et al. Natural history of acute coronary heart attacks. A community study. *Br Heart J* 1972; **34**: 67-80.

2. Piza Z. Sudden death: A world-wide problem. In: Kulbertus HE, Wellens HJJ, eds. *Sudden Death*. The Hague: Martinus Nijhoff, 1980: 3-10.

3. Kuller L, Cooper M, Perper J. Epidemiology of sudden death. *Arch Intern Med* 1972; **129**: 714-9.

4. Oliver MFL. Home or hospital for acute myocardial infarction? *Lancet* 1978; i: 1089.

5. Thompson RG, Hallstrom AP, Cobb LA. Bystander-initiated cardiopulmonary resuscitation in the management of ventricular fibrillation. *Ann Intern Med* 1979; **90**: 737-40.

6. Mackintosh AF, Crabb ME, Grainger R, Williams JM, Chamberlain DA. The Brighton Resuscitation Ambulances: Review of forty consecutive survivors of out-of-hospital cardiac arrest. *Br Med J* 1978; **1**: 1115-8.

7. Hampton JR, Dowling M, Nichols C. Comparison of results from a cardiac ambulance manned by medical or non-medical personnel. *Lancet* 1977; i: 526-9.

8. Di Francesco D, Ojeda C. Properties of the current if in the sinoatrial node of the rabbit compared with those of the current $^ik_2$ in Purkinje fibres. *J Physiol* 1980; **308**: 353-67.

9. Yanagihara K, Irisawa H. Potassium current during pacemaker depolarization in the rabbit sinotrial node cells. *Pflügers Arch* 1980; **388**: 255-60.

10. Sheridan DJ, Penkoske PA, Sobel BE, Corr PB. Alpha-adrenergic contributions to dysrhythmia during myocardial ischaemia and reperfusion in cats. *J Clin Invest* 1980; **65**: 161-71.

11. Cranfield PF, Wit AL, Hoffman BF. Genesis of cardiac arrhythmias. *Circulation* 1973; **47**: 190-204.

12. Ferrier GR, Saunders JH, Mendez CA. A cellular mechanism for the generation of ventricular arrhythmias by acetylstrophanthidin. *Circ Res* 1973; **32**: 600-9.

13. Kass RS, Tsien RW, Weingart R. Ionic basis of transient inward current induced by strophanthidin in cardiac Purkinje fibres. *J Physiol (Lond)* 1978; **281**: 209-26.

14. Kimura S, Cameron J, Kozlovskis P, Bassett A, Myerburg R. Delayed after-depolarisations and triggered activity induced in feline Purkinje fibres by alpha-adrenergic stimulation in the presence of elevated calcium levels. *Circulation* 1984; **70**: 1074-82.

15. Mines GR. On dynamic equilibrium in the heart. *J Physiol (Lond)* 1913; **46**: 349-82.

16. Allessie MA, Banke FIM, Schopman FLG. Circus movement in rabbit atrial muscle as a mechanism of tachycardia. III. The 'leading circle' concept: A new model of circus movement in cardiac tissue without the involvement of an anatomical obstacle. *Circ Res* 1977; **41**: 9-18.

17. Penny WJ, Sheridan DJ. Arrhythmias and cellular electrophysiological changes during myocardial ischaemia and reper-fusion. *Cardiovasc Res* 1983; **17**: 363-72.

18. Kleber AG. Resting membrane potential, extracellular potassium activity and intracellular sodium activity during acute global ischaemia in isolated perfused guinea-pig hearts. *Circ Res* 1986; **52**: 442-50.

19. Meesmann W. Early arrhythmias and primary ventricular fibrillation after acute myocardial ischaemia in relation to pre-existing coronary collaterals. In: Parratt J, ed. *Early Arrhythmias Resulting from Myocardial Ischaemia*. London: Macmillan, 1982; 93-112.

20. Hirche H, Franz C, Bos L, Bissig R, Lang R, Schramm M. Myocardial extracellular K+ and H+ increase and noradrenaline release as possible cause of early arrhythmias following acute coronary artery occlusion in pigs. *J Mol Cell Cardiol* 1980; **12**: 579-93.

21. Parratt JR. Inhibitors of the slow calcium current and early ventricular arrhythmias. In: Parratt JR, ed. *Early Arrhythmias Resulting from Myocardial Ischaemia*. London: Macmillan, 1982: 327-46.

22. Cohnheim J, Von Schulthess-Rechberg A. Über die folgen der Kranzarterien verschleissung für das Herz. *Virchows Arch* 1881; **85**: 503-37.

23. Araki HJ, Koiwaya J, Nakagaki O, Nakamuna M. Diurnal distribution of ST segment elevation and related arrhythmias in patients with variant angina. *Circulation* 1983; **67**: 995-1000.

24. Previtali M, Klersy C, Salerno JA. Ventricular tachyarrhythmias in Prinzmetal's variant angina: Chemical significance and relation to the degree and time course of ST segment elevation. *Am J Cardiol* 1983; **52**: 19-25.

25. Penny WJ, Culling W, Lewis MJ, Sheridan DJ. Antiarrhythmic and electrophysiological effects of alpha-adrenoceptor blockade during myocardial ischaemia and reperfusion in isolated guinea-pig heart. *J Mol Cell Cardiol* 1985; **17**: 399-409.

26. Culling W, Penny WJ, Lewis MJ, Middleton K, SheridanDJ. Effects of myocardial catecholamine depletion on cellular electrophysiology and arrhythmias during ischaemia and reperfusion. *Cardiovasc Res* 1984; **18**: 675-82.

27. Davies MJ. Pathological view of sudden death. *Br Heart J* 1981; **45**: 88-96.

28. Friedman PL, Stewart JR, Wit AL. Survival of subendocardial Purkinje fibres after extensive myocardial infarction in dogs. *Circ Res* 1973; **33**: 597-611.

29. Lazzara R, El-Sherif M, Sherlag BJ. Early and late effects of coronary occlusion on canine Purkinje fibres. *Circ Res* 1974; **35**: 391-9.

30. Myerburg RJ, Bassett AL, Epstein K, et al.Electrophysiological effects of procainamide in acute and healed experimental ischaemic injury in cat myocardium. *Circ Res* 1982; **50**: 386-93.

31. Garan H, Fallon JI, Ruskin JN. Sustained ventricular tachycardia in recent myocardial infarction. *Circulation* 1980; **62**: 980-7.

32. Michelson EL, Spear JR, Moore EN. Electrophysiology and anatomic correlates of sustained ventricular tachyarrhythmias in a model of chronic myocardial infarction. *Am J Cardiol* 1980; **45**: 483-590.

33. Horowitz LN, Harken AM, Kastor JA, Josephson ME. Ventricular resection guided by epicardial and endocardial mapping for treatment of recurrent ventricular tachycardia. *N Engl J Med* 1980; **302**: 589-93.

34. Nathan AW. Surgery for the treatment of tachycardias. In: Camm AJ, Ward DE, eds. *Clinical Aspects of Cardiac Arrhythmias.* Lancaster: Kluwer Academic Publishers, 1988; 375-401.

35. Riemersma RA. Myocardial catecholamine release in acute ischaemia; Relationship to cardiac arrhythmias. In: Parratt JR, ed. *Early Arrhythmias Resulting from Myocardial Ischaemia.* London: Macmillan, 1982; 125-38.

36. Sheridan DJ. Myocardial alpha-adrenoceptors and arrhythmias induced by myocardial ischaemia. In: Parratt JR, ed. *Early Arrhythmias Resulting from Myocardial Ischaemia.* London: Macmillan, 1982; 317-29.

37. Nazum FR, Bischoff F. Urinary output of catechol derivatives including adrenaline in normal individuals in essential hypertension and myocardial infaction. *Circulation* 1953; **7**: 96-101.

38. Gazes PC, Richardson JA, Woods EF. Plasma catecholamine concentrations in myocardial infarction and angina pectoris. *Circulation* 1959; **19**: 657-61.

39. Wollenberger A, Shahab L. Anoxia-induced release of noradrenaline from the isolated perfused heart. *Nature (Lond)* 1965; **207**: 88-9.

40. Guaduel Y, Karaguenzian HS, DeLeiris J. Deleterious effects of endogenous catecholamines on hypoxic myocardial cells following re-oxygenation. *J Mol Cell Cardiol* 1979; **11**: 717-31.

41. Sethi V, Haider B, Ahmed S, Oldwurstel HA, Regan TJ.Influence of B-blockade and chemical sympathectomy on myocardial function and arrhythmias in acute ischaemia. *Cardiovasc Res* 1973; **7**: 740-7.

42. Ebert PA, Vanderbeck RB, Allgood RJ, Sabiston DC. Effect of chronic cardiac denervation on arrhythmias after coronary artery ligation. *Cardiovasc Res* 1970; **4**: 141-7.

43. Lombardi F, Verrier RL, Lown B. Relationship between sympathetic neural activity, coronary dynamics and vulnerability to ventricular fibrillation during myocardial ischaemia and reperfusion. *Am Heart J* 1983; **105**: 958-65.

44. Fitzgerald JA. The effects of B-adrenoceptor blocking drugs on early arrhythmias in experimental and clinical myocardial ischaemia. In: Parratt JR, ed. *Early Arrhythmias Resulting from Myocardial Ischaemia.* London: Macmillan, 1982; 295-316.

45. Beta-blocker Heart Attack Trials Research Group. A randomized trial of propranolol in patients with acute myocardial infarctions. *JAMA* 1982; **247**: 1707-14.

46. Baber NS. Primary and secondary prevention of coronary artery disease by drug therapy. In: Breckenridge A, ed. *Drugs in the Management of Heart Disease.* Lancaster: MTP Press, 1985; 79-159.

47. Stewart JR, Burmeister WE, Burmeister J, Lucchesi BR. Electrophysiologic and antiarrhythmic effects of phentolamine in experimental coronary artery occlusion and reperfusion in the dog. *J Cardiovasc Pharmacol* 1980; **2**: 77-91.

48. Mathes P, Gudbjarnason S. Changes in norepinephrine stores in the canine heart following experimental myocardial infarction. *Am Heart J* 1971; **81**: 211-9.

49. Verrier RL, Hohnloser SH. How is the nervous system implicated in the genesis of cardiac arrhythmias? In: Hearse DJ, Manning AS, Janse MJ, eds. *Life-threatening Arrhythmias during Ischaemia and Infarction.* New York: Raven Press, 1987; 153-68.

50. Culling W, Penny WJ, Cunliffe G, Flores NA, Sheridan DJ. Arrhythmogenic and electrophysiological effects of alpha-adrenoceptor stimulation during myocardial ischaemia and reperfusion. *J Mol Cell Cardiol* 1987; **19**: 251-8.

51. Corr B, Shayman JA, Kramer JB, Kipnis RJ. Alpha-adrenoceptor receptors in ischaemic cat myocardium. A potential mediator of electrophysiological derangements. *J Clin Invest* 1981; **67**: 1232-6.

52. Crome R, Hearse DJ, Maguire ME, Manning AS. Dissociation between reperfusion arrhythmias and increases in ventricular alpha-receptor density in the anaesthetized rat. *Br J Pharmacol* 1985; **86**: 498.

53. Broadley KJ, Chess-Williams RG, Sheridan DJ. [3H]-prazosin binding during ischaemia and reperfusion in the guinea-pig Langendorff heart. *Br J Pharmacol* 1985; **86**: 759.

54. Aubry ML, Davey MJ, Petch B. UK-52,046 – A novel alpha$_1$-adrenoceptor antagonist with antidysrhythmic activity. *Br J Pharmacol* 1988; **95**: 752.

55. Harris AS, Toth LA, Hoey TE. Arrhythmic and antiarrhythmic effects of sodium, potassium, and calcium salts and of glucose injected into coronary arteries of infarcted and normal hearts. *Circulation* 1958; **1**: 1318-28.

56. Benzing H, Strohm M, Gebert G. The effect of local ischaemia on the ionic activity of dog myocardial interstitium. In: Betz E, ed. *Vascular Smooth Muscle.* Berlin: Springer-Verlag, 1972; 172-4.

57. Gettes LS. Electrophysiological basis of arrhythmias in acute myocardial ischaemia. In: Oliver MF, ed. *Modern Trends in Cardiology, Vol. 3.* London: Butterworth, 1974; 219-46.

58. Hirche H, Friedrich R, Kebbel U, McDonald F, Zylka V. Early arrhythmias, myocardial extracellular potassium and pH. In: Parratt JR, ed. *Early Arrhythmias Resulting from Myocardial Ischaemia.* London: Macmillan, 1982; 113-24.

59. Gettes L. What are the effects of potassium on the electrophysiology of acute ischaemia? In: Hearse DJ, Manning AS, Janse MJ, eds. *Life-threatening Arrhythmias during Ischaemia and Infarction.* New York: Raven Press, 1987; 77-8.

60. Russell D. Early ventricular arrhythmias: Relationship of electrophysiology to blood flow and metabolism. In: Parratt JR, ed. *Early Arrhythmias Resulting from Myocardial Ischaemia.* London: Macmillan, 1982; 37-56.

61. Hill JL, Gettes LS. Effect of acute coronary artery occlusion on local myocardial extracellular K+ activity in swine. *Circulation* 1980; **61**: 770-8.

62. Woodward B, Manning AS. Reperfusion arrhythmias: Are free radicals involved? In: Hearse DJ, Manning AS, Janse MJ, eds. *Life-threatening Arrhythmias during Ischaemia and Infarction.* New York: Raven Press, 1987; 115-33.

63. Bernier M, Hearse DJ, Manning AS. Reperfusion-induced arrhythmias and oxygen-derived free radicals. Studies with anti-free radical interventions and a free radical generating system in the isolated

perfused rat heart. *Circ Res* 1986; **58**: 331-40.

64. Rosen R, Dansch W, Beck E, Klaus W. Platelet-induced aggravation of acute ischaemia in an isolated rabbit heart model. *Cardiovasc Res* 1987; **21**: 293-8.

65. Kammermeir H, Ober M. Essential contribution of thrombocytes to the occurrence of catecholamine-induced cardiac necrosis. *J Mol Cell Cardiol* 1985; **17**: 371-6.

66. Chakrabarty S, Thomas P, Williams T, Sheridan DJ. Influence of platelets on extent of myocardial infarction during coronary artery occlusion. *Br Heart J* 1989; **61(1)**: 78.

67. Golino P, Ashton JH, Maximillian B, et al. Local platelet activation causes vasoconstriction of large epicardial canine coronary arteries in vivo. *Circulation* 1989; **79**: 154-66.

68. El-Sharic N, Myerburg RJ, Scherlag BJ, et al. Electrocardiographic antecedents of primary ventricular fibrillation. *Br Heart J* 1976; **38**: 415-22.

69. Lown B, Fakhro AM, Hood WB, Thorn GW. The coronary care unit. New perspectives and directions. *JAMA* 1967; **19**: 188-9.

70. Campbell RWF, Murray A, Julian DG. Ventricular arrhythmias in first 12 hours of acute myocardial infarction. Natural history study. *Br Heart J* 1981; **46**: 351-7.

71. Dubois C, Smeets JP, Demoulin C, et al. Incidence, clinical significance and prognosis of ventricular fibrillation in the early phase of myocardial infarction. *Eur Heart J* 1986; **7**: 945-51.

72. Lie KI, Wellens HJJ, Von Capelle FJ, Durrer D. Lidocaine in the prevention of primary ventricular fibrillation. *N Engl J Med* 1974; **29**: 1324-6.

73. Goldberg R, Szklo M, Tonascia J, Kennedy HL. Acute myocardial infarction. Prognosis complicated by ventricular fibrillation or cardiac arrest. *JAMA* 1979; **241**: 2024-7.